How To Keep Your Teeth
For A Lifetime

How To Keep Your Teeth For A Lifetime

✦

What You Should Know About Caring For Your Teeth

B. Theo Clifford

iUniverse, Inc.
Bloomington

How to Keep Your Teeth for a Lifetime
What You Should Know About Caring for Your Teeth

iUniverse books may be ordered through booksellers or by contacting:

iUniverse
1663 Liberty Drive
Bloomington, IN 47403
www.iuniverse.com
1-800-Authors (1-800-288-4677)

ISBN: 978-1-4759-6450-9 (sc)
ISBN: 978-1-4759-6452-3 (hc)
ISBN: 978-1-4759-6451-6 (ebk)

Printed in the United States of America

iUniverse rev. date: 12/17/2012

In loving memory of my parents and to the wonderful woman who has stood beside me for over 44 years as my wife.

You only have to take care of the teeth you want to keep!

Robert "Bob" Allen, Hygienist, MSGT, USAF Retired

CONTENTS

ILLUSTRATIONS

PREFACE

On occasion if we are paying attention to the news, we learn from the World Health Organization that 60-90% of school children and nearly 100% of adults have dental cavities.[1] Why, with all of the advancements in dentistry, is tooth decay still a leading disease in the world? It is my belief that it is caused first and foremost by a widespread lack of education about how to correctly take care of our teeth and the very vital role our teeth have in our overall good health.

During my twenty plus years experience in dentistry, I have been surprised at the lack of knowledge people have about their teeth and how to properly care for them. I am amazed to see so many people with teeth missing or wearing dentures. Then I think back on how I was raised and I realize why. My parents and grandparents never knew anything about how to properly care for their teeth so they could not instruct me to properly take care of mine. They were all plagued with dental problems and ended up with missing teeth and dentures. In my early school years I was taught only to brush my teeth and even then *I was taught incorrectly*. I learned some things from the advertisements for different dental products, but that was confusing sometimes and left me with questions about which products were really the best, necessary or how to use them correctly. I read very few articles written about dental problems because I didn't think they would ever apply to me. When I visited a dentist for the first time at about the age of 9, it was to have an abscessed tooth pulled and it was a very bad experience for me. The next time I visited a dentist at about age 16, I needed a great deal

---

[1]   World Health Organization, Oral health. Fact sheet No 318, April 2012

of dental work done including having another abscessed tooth pulled. Believe me I did not spend a lot of time asking my dentist questions, I just wanted him to fix my problems and let me out of there. Like most of you, I did not like being there. Do you recognize any of my reasons for not knowing more? Have you had the same kind of experiences?

I have talked with many people who just like me did not know how to take care of their teeth and in many cases were taught the wrong things resulting in the loss of their teeth. In most cases they also paid a big price in dollars. *This does not need to happen!* This is part of the reason I decided to write this book; to help inform those who want to be informed. Many people want to take care of their teeth but have been given no information or given the wrong information. They will never get their dental condition completely under control until they get the right information. Please realize that there is a way to stop tooth decay. The more we know the less it will affect us and our families.

Another big reason for our poor dental condition is our acceptance of tooth decay as a normal part of life. We have acquired the attitude that decay is acceptable; that everyone has decay and so decay is a natural part of our lives. We accept that our grandparents had dentures and so did our parents and *we will also*! We do not believe that we can do much to prevent decay and instead accept it as a normal consequence of our inaction. We are raised to accept defeat because we have adapted to the loss of our teeth and do not recognize it as a major life changing loss. It is with these reasons in mind that I write this book.

In writing this book I have drawn from my experience of over 20 years of working in dentistry. I am not a dentist; however I have worked as a dental hygienist, dental assistant and an expanded functions dental assistant. I have worked with over 80 different dentists. Part of what I have learned from them I am passing on to you. This book will give you some basic guidance and the insight necessary to help you keep your teeth. You will not need a background in dentistry to understand this book. This book is written in a very basic and simplistic way and in language that should be easily understood. I have tried to write this book as if I had you as a patient and was explaining to you the different ways of caring for your teeth. This book will give you the necessary knowledge and tools to correctly care for your teeth and help you avoid the pitfalls that cause or contribute to tooth decay and eventually the loss of your teeth.

It is very important that you understand that what I have written in this book are my own ideas taken from the experience I have had with those dentists I have worked with and from the patients I have worked on. This book and my opinions are not intended to replace appropriate dental advice and treatment from your dentist. I do not know all the information necessary for every problem there is which will involve the mouth. Your dentist is still the best one to seek out for information. I want to give you enough information so you will be able to ask good questions and know which direction you should be going then recognize it when you hear it from your dentist. Always remember that the choice is yours about the level of care you want to have. You are the one who decides to take care of your teeth or to neglect them. The majority of your dental problems will be created and controlled by you. You can have what ever you are willing to work for; that's the bottom line.

I have included in the back of this book a glossary of terms that may be unfamiliar to you and I have also included footnotes to assist you. Some of these footnotes are examples of various dental products and locations for services and *are highlighted as examples*. Because a product or location is mentioned in this book does not imply an endorsement of that product or location. It is listed simply as an example to let you know that these products and locations do exist and that is there only purpose for being mentioned.

Please understand that this book is intended to be an informative resource and not an authoritative resource. It is not all inclusive and it will not tell you everything that can happen to your teeth. Additionally, recognize that each person is different and that while we may all have similarities, what may happen to one person, may not happen to another. This book is not intended to replace your need to seek proper dental care from dental professionals and to follow their guidance. I hope you not only learn from this book, but will pass this information on to those you care about.

ACKNOWLEDGMENTS

First and foremost I must acknowledge the timeless efforts of my editor, Tami who took my jumbled thoughts and helped me organize them into something understandable.

I also want to add that this book is possible only because of the dedicated dentist I have had the privilege of working with. I will not name all of them, but a few of them took the time and had the patience to help me learn more about dentistry and in particular their specialized areas. I want to thank Mike Brunsvold, Ralph Lambert, Norm Savers, William Assiker, Danny Crout, Mark Eggert, Patrick Domine and Marlin Montgomery. Each of these dentists left an impression on me and it is because of them that I was able to compile this book.

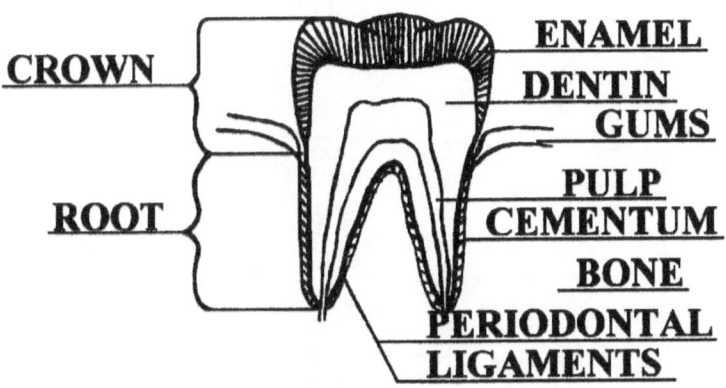

Anatomy of a tooth and surrounding tissues
(Refer to this illustration as you read this book.)

BRUSHING YOUR TEETH

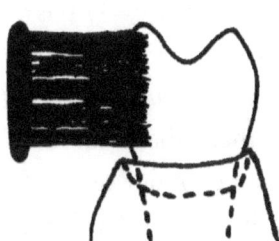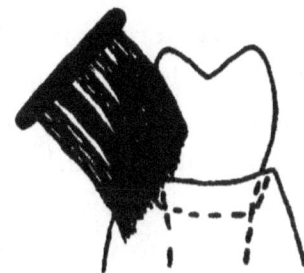

Holding your toothbrush flat against your teeth will only allow you to clean your teeth and not the area below the gum line. Holding your toothbrush at a 45 degree angle will allow you to brush your teeth, get the bristles under the gum line and clean the sulcus. You will also massage the gum tissue at the same time. The results are healthier teeth and gums.

Brushing your teeth is the heart of good oral hygiene. It is the single most important thing you can do to protect your teeth, gums and overall oral health. How frequently you brush your teeth is very important. I know you have heard the common instruction to "brush your teeth after every meal and whenever you eat anything." We have been taught this by our parents, teachers, dentists and everyone else. If you have developed a habit of brushing two, or three times a day, do not stop. Keep up the good work! If you have not, do not feel guilty or feel that you are a bad parent if your children don't. In my opinion it is not totally necessary. Now please don't stop reading here, you must hear me out! The following is probably information that you may have never heard before.

Why do we brush

We brush to remove food particles and bacteria. Food particles and bacteria are the causes of plaque, tartar (calculus), decay, gum disease (periodontal disease) and of course bad breath. There are other things that contribute also, but I'll stay with the things that are most common.

When we eat, we coat our teeth with food particles. This is especially true of sticky foods. These particles combine with bacteria and saliva in our mouth and become plaque. *Plaque is a major cause of dental problems.* Plaque is a soft, sticky substance that adheres to our teeth and produces an acid that stays next to the enamel of our teeth. When left on our teeth for over twelve plus hours, it starts to harden and form tartar (calculus).[2] It attacks our teeth and gums and starts its destructive process. If it is removed during this twelve plus hour period, the cycle is stopped and must be started over. Therefore it is only necessary to brush at least once a day. However, your brushing must be completely effective if you are going to brush only once in a twelve hour period.

It is unlikely that a person will do an effective job of brushing in 1 to 3 minutes a day. If you think you can then you probably have dental problems. To be effective, you will need to spend more time just brushing. To be thorough takes time. As long as I can remember there has been an acceptable time of 2 to 3 minutes spent on brushing by an adult, usually less for a child. The makers of dental products are trying to get you to brush more effectively in those 2 to 3 minutes rather than to brush longer. That is the driving force behind many of the different styles of toothbrushes and mechanical devices available on the market. If you brush effectively in those 2 to 3 minutes, keep at it. However the best thing to do is to increase the amount of time spent brushing.

In my opinion if you brush only once a day then it must be after your last meal or snack and before you go to bed. Think about it. If

---

[2]   TLC for gums Therapeutic Laser Care, www.TLC4Gums.com

you brush only in the morning, food particles and bacteria are on your teeth for approximately 24 hours. If you brush before bed, these same particles are only on your teeth from when you eat in the morning until you brush at night. This reduces the opportunity for dental problems to begin. Parents that have their children brush before going to bed are on the right track.

Most of us do not want to stand at a sink for 5 to 10 minutes brushing our teeth. Consequently, we will not develop a habit of doing this. I would recommend that you brush (without toothpaste) while watching TV, reading a book, studying, or working on a computer. That is what I do, however, I do not do it when in a restaurant, working or driving. I have done this for many years with great results. Although I've had a lot of dental work done because of neglect while I was young, I haven't had any new decay for the past 40 years because of neglect. Additionally, my gums do not bleed and are in excellent shape. The bone support for my teeth is outstanding.

When I brush this way without toothpaste, I swallow my saliva. I swallow it all day long anyway so it's not any different. I just had to mentally get use to it. I take the time to brush each tooth and spend the time necessary to get it clean. I do it unconsciously because I'm doing other things and I don't rush through it. My teeth really do feel nice and clean when I'm finished. Another benefit I received is that brushing my teeth helps me to stay awake and alert. It may do the same for you.

Although I do not use toothpaste at the above mentioned times, it is still necessary to rinse my toothbrush each time I finish. If I didn't rinse my toothbrush, I would be using a toothbrush that would contain food debris and bacteria which had been growing since last used. This would be reintroduced into my mouth. That's a way of causing new problems. A rule to follow: Always rinse your toothbrush before and after use.

The time you invest in brushing will generate a greater benefit if you are brushing correctly. When I was a child, I was taught to hold my toothbrush flat against my teeth and sweep it towards the top or biting surface of my teeth. I was brushing my teeth but not cleaning the area around each tooth next to the gum line. We all have a small open area around each tooth, next to the gum line. *It is called the sulcus.* This is where debris and bacteria are trapped and begin to cause damage. Because I did not know better, I brushed this way for almost twenty years and consequently because I was brushing incorrectly, I have the fillings to prove it. I also had problems with my gums bleeding. I was 25 years old before I learned how to correctly take care of my teeth. Realize it doesn't matter how old you are, you can still learn to correctly take care of your teeth.

Let me make some recommendations for brushing correctly. First, use a soft or extra soft bristled toothbrush. Hold your toothbrush at an angle (about 45 degrees) so the bristles will go underneath your gum tissue into the sulcus. Use a gentle back and forth or circular motion as you brush. You want to get the bristles of your toothbrush under your gum tissue so it can remove the bacteria and debris. This will also remove any plaque on your teeth, all in one motion. Take time to clean as much of the area between your teeth as you can reach with your toothbrush. Do this on all of your teeth; front, back, on top and behind your back teeth.

The areas where plaque turns into tartar the fastest are on the outside of your top molars and on the inside of your lower front teeth. This occurs because these are the areas where saliva enters your mouth and mixes with plaque to form tartar. Because of this fact, you should spend more time brushing these areas.

If you are not sure if you are doing a thorough job of brushing, try using a disclosing tablet or mouth rinse. It is what your dentist or hygienist has you use and then spit out to show what areas you are missing with your toothbrush. You can purchase them at your local drugstore or market. They are a great help if you are trying to get younger children to brush correctly. Be careful when you have them spit it out though. Depending on what type you give them, it can be a mess to cleanup.

If your gum tissue is unhealthy, it may bleed for a while when you begin brushing this way (see the section on bleeding gums). After you have brushed correctly for several weeks and used your dental floss, (see the next section), you will notice your teeth and gums feel better and the bleeding should be stopped. If the bleeding has not stopped, see your dentist. You may need additional help.

If you have difficulty brushing your teeth and getting under your gums, you may want to concentrate on doing each tooth separately until you can do it automatically. The important thing is that each area must be cleaned daily. It does not depend on which type of brush stroke you use, back and forth, circular or a combination of the two. What's important is that you clean each area thoroughly.

FLOSSING

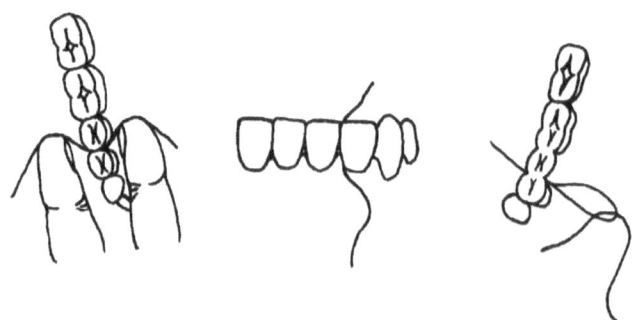

If your teeth are close together, you cannot get your toothbrush between your teeth. You must use dental floss if you want to clean these areas. Wrap your floss around your middle finger (or two fingers) and leave yourself about 1 inch between your fingers to floss with. Push the floss back, away from, the area you are flossing. This will allow the floss to slide into the sulcus and not cut your gum tissue. Your floss will go below your gum tissue into the sulcus around each tooth and not hurt you. However if you take it down to far, you could cause some pain and damage, so be careful. By using a floss threader, you can get the floss under your bridge if you have one. It is vital these teeth be flossed as well as all others.

The purpose of dental floss is very misunderstood. Dental floss is not something to use just when you get something caught between your teeth or when you need extra strong string. Although it does have many uses, it is designed to remove food and plaque from between your teeth and below your gum tissue. Flossing, along with brushing properly, is the most important thing you can do to keep your teeth and gums healthy.

The value of flossing must not be overlooked or underestimated. We are all aware of the importance of brushing our teeth because it has been drilled into us by our parents, teachers, dentist, and the mass media. However, little is said about flossing and yet, it is just as important as brushing if not more important. The value of flossing cannot be stressed enough. If you get your teeth cleaned by a hygienist, they may show you how to floss your teeth. Hopefully, they will also tell you what will happen if you do not floss.

Rarely are we given an explanation of why flossing is necessary. When you brush your teeth you brush 3 sides: the front, the back, and the top. But what about the two surfaces between your teeth? There are still 2 surfaces which for most of us, our toothbrushes will not reach very well. It is vital that these surfaces be cleaned as well. Many of our cavities start between the teeth where the toothbrush will not reach. Floss will reach these areas and it will clean effectively if done correctly.

Fighting tooth decay is not the main reason I feel so strongly about flossing. The main reason is periodontal disease. I have seen people with beautiful teeth, who have no decay but still they lose their teeth. This is because of periodontal disease. Many people think that because their parents lost their teeth when they were young (between 30 and 45) they will too. *That may be the case, but it does not have to be.* In most cases, you should be able to keep your teeth throughout your life if you keep them clean. This takes more than just brushing.

Let me explain. As we eat and drink, tiny food particles get trapped between our teeth and under our gums. If they are not removed daily, they begin to form plaque that attacks the tooth structure and gums. As it attacks the gum tissue, the gums may get infected or very red and bleed easily when brushed. There may be tenderness and slight swelling. These are the first signs of gum disease or periodontal disease. If you catch it right away and use correct brushing and flossing techniques combined with rinsing your mouth with warm saltwater, you may stop the symptoms yourself in a couple of weeks. You should still have a dentist check you over and have your gums and bone condition evaluated. This condition known as gum disease or gingivitis will be discussed more in the section on periodontal disease.

If you are a beginner at using floss, I recommend that you use waxed floss or one of the types that slides easily between your teeth. There is a reduced chance of damage to your gum tissue while you are learning to maneuver your fingers inside your mouth. The waxed floss does give off a small wax residue, however it is not harmful and you will probably not notice it. If you have teeth that are close together, this type of floss is best because they will slide through the contacts points better. When you get more adept at using floss, you may want to switch to non-waxed type of floss. Both types clean very effectively.

Floss is available in many different sizes. There is fine non-waxed floss which can be used between teeth that are close together, medium sized floss, and what is called dental tape or wide waxed floss. If you have an advanced periodontal condition or large spaces between your teeth, you may want to try using what is called dental ribbon. It is floss with a yarn attached. It has the advantage of covering and polishing a large area very quickly. It should only be used when there is a wide space between the teeth.

How do you use floss

There are several methods for using floss, but I will give you the one I find works best. Because you will be placing your fingers in your mouth, I recommend washing your hands before you start. Take a piece of floss about 24 inches long and wrap it around your two middle fingers, leaving your index fingers free. I recommend using two fingers instead of one so it does not cut off your blood circulation so much. Keep an eye on your finger tips and if they are turning blue, loosen your floss. Wrap it around the fingers several times, enough to keep the floss from sliding free. Wrap the remainder of the floss around the two middle fingers on the other hand. Let out enough floss that you can hold it by applying pressure against it with your index fingers and your thumbs, and have about 1 inch between them (refer to the illustration). As you use the floss you will unwrap it from one hand and wrap it up on the other, thus giving yourself fresh floss when you want it.

Sometimes it is easier to use a mirror when you begin flossing, but you should work at being able to do it without a mirror. You will have to put your fingers inside your mouth to floss correctly and you will use your index fingers and thumbs together, depending upon which teeth you are flossing. Begin by gently sliding the floss between your teeth. Do not snap it between your teeth because you could damage your gum tissue. After you have the floss between your teeth, put your fingers back, or away from the tooth you are flossing. This will wrap the floss around the tooth surface you are going to floss (refer to the illustration). Gently move the floss up and down several times or until the tooth feels clean. It may take some time before you will feel the difference, but it will come. Be sure to take the floss below the gums next to the tooth. This is the space where the gums are unattached to the teeth, or the sulcus. It is vital that this area be cleaned and is one of the main reasons you should floss your teeth. Take the floss as far down as you can without hurting your gums. Do this with every tooth. Do it on teeth that do not have an adjacent tooth next to them and behind your back teeth.

Sometimes when you are flossing and getting your floss under the gum line as you should, you may not be able to get it back up. You may have very tight contacts, a filling between your teeth with an overhang on it, or perhaps you have a crown that the margins hang over a little. It is important that you do not try to pull your floss back up through the contacts. You could pull the crown off, dislodge the filling, or break off the floss between your teeth and not be able to get it out. If you break it off, try using another piece of waxed floss to dislodge it. If you get it through, do not pull it back up. Instead, release the floss from one of your hands and pull it out rather than up. Keep flossing those areas as they will need it even more than other areas. If you get it stuck and cannot dislodge it with your floss, see your dentist and let them dislodge it. Do not try everything you can think of to dislodge it yourself as you could do a lot of damage.

If you are unable to use your fingers inside your mouth, do not give up. There are floss aids which will do the job for you and they work very effectively.[3] They are very good if you are flossing the teeth of someone else such as an elderly or disabled person, or younger children. These people need their teeth flossed also and it will save you additional dental bills if you take the time to do it. Teach them to do it if possible.

If you have a bridge in your mouth, you must floss under it. If you don't, you will develop periodontal disease under the bridge. In time you will lose the bridge and possibly your teeth as well. This can be avoided and the bridge maintained very easily with the use of a device called a floss threader.[4] There are several types of floss threaders made from plastic and wire. They operate by the same principle as a needle and thread. Thread the floss through the end of the floss threader and then run the floss threader under your bridge. Floss the teeth at both ends of your bridge and run it along the bridge to remove any buildup it may have. It is a simple thing to do but it can have some very bad consequences if you neglect to do it.

When should you floss

I am often asked when the best time is to floss and how often it should be done. *Flossing should be done daily.* The best time is whenever you can fit it in and make it a habit. You will want to have about 5 minutes available after you become proficient. I recommend doing it at night before going to bed. Do it when brushing your teeth. Not everyone will have the same schedule, but do it sometime during the day.

---

3   Example: Plackers, Ranir, LLC, www.plackers.com
4   Example: GUM Eez-Thru Floss Threader, Sunstar Americas, Inc. GUMbrand.com

It is best to use a mirror when you start learning to floss. When you can, stop using the mirror. This will allow you the freedom of being able to floss somewhere other than in your bathroom. My best time to floss is when I am watching TV, reading or working at my computer. I am not limited in time and I can do as thorough a flossing as I want to. I also use a flossing aid so that I only have to put my fingers in my mouth to floss under my bridge. This frees up one hand to do other things. No matter how you choose to floss, the important thing is that you floss your teeth daily. If you cannot do it for five minutes, do it for as long as you can, *but do it*!

TOOTHBRUSHES

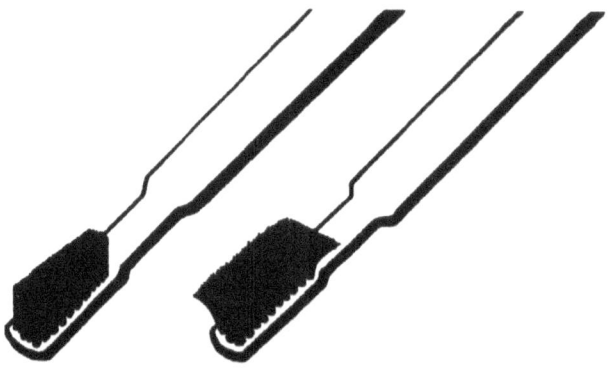

A toothbrush is the most important instrument for proper oral hygiene. The size and shape are not as important as that it has soft bristles and is used regularly. When your toothbrush begins to flare out, it is time to replace it with a new toothbrush.

As you might expect, I have definite ideas about what type of toothbrush is best. When I was young, I would only buy hard toothbrushes. I liked that I could get one to last for almost a year. I also felt that I was getting my teeth very clean because the bristles were so stiff. Well, thank goodness I later learned differently. The only toothbrush I will use now and recommend is a soft or extra soft toothbrush. Hard and medium toothbrushes have their place and if you like them, use them. For me their place is cleaning the tile in the bathroom or around the windows or similar things. Never will I put them in my mouth again. Hard and medium brushes do not have the flexibility to get between your teeth and under your gum tissue into the sulcus. These types of brushes can also tear up your gum tissue. This is part of the reason why people end up with gum disease. You can look in a mirror and see stains between your teeth where a hard or medium toothbrush cannot reach. You can also easily tell that your brush, or the way you use it, is not doing all it should. Check your brush and the brushing method you use. You should be able to keep your teeth free from most stains if you're brushing correctly.

Is the style of toothbrush important

The style of toothbrush you use is not as vital as the softness of the bristles. Choose a straight one or one with the bent head or any of the new combinations, whichever type you prefer. All of them should perform as they are designed to. What matters is that you feel comfortable with what you use, and that you use it often. I do have my favorite style, and although I've tried many of the new styles, I still prefer my favorite, you may as well.

Toothbrushes should be replaced about every 3 months. If you notice the bristles on your toothbrush have started to fan out, it is time to change it. Keep an eye on your children's toothbrushes as well and change them when needed.

If you have been using a hard or medium toothbrush, you may not think you are cleaning your teeth when you switch to a soft toothbrush. Continue with the soft toothbrush and you should notice a big difference before too long. You will most likely never go back to the hard or medium brush.

It is important that you keep your toothbrush clean. Rinse it after each use. Store it in an area where it can be kept separate from other toothbrushes, especially if anyone in your household is sick. If your toothbrush is kept in a bathroom, it is advised that it be kept as far away as possible from your toilet because of the aerosol that is created each time the toilet is flushed. That aerosol has the potential of containing many germs.

MECHANICAL TOOTHBRUSHES AND IRRIGATION DEVICES

I am sold on brushing your teeth with a good toothbrush and taking the time to do the job right. But what about using powered toothbrushes? I have some concerns about using them. It's not the toothbrushes I'm concerned about. Toothbrushes do what they are designed to do. I'm concerned about the user. Often when a person uses a powered toothbrush, they do not take the time to do a thorough job of brushing. As stated previously we spend an acceptable average of two to three minutes or less brushing our teeth. Using a powered toothbrush may make those two to three minutes more effective but only if it is done correctly. However, most people like to take shortcuts. If you skimp on your brushing even using a powered brush, you may have the misconception of thinking you are doing enough when you may not be. I have some concerns with that and you should too.

Another concern is that if your powered toothbrush is weak or out of power completely, you won't brush effectively and spend the time needed to do a thorough job. If your children use only the powered toothbrush and do not know how to effectively clean their teeth with a regular toothbrush, you could be creating future problems for them and yourself.

I wholeheartedly support using a powered toothbrush by those who have a disability or handicap that prevents them from using a regular toothbrush. It's the best thing to do to assist them especially since they need extra attention paid to their oral hygiene.

If you choose to use a powered toothbrush, I suggest one that rotates the bristles or goes back and forth, but not up and down. This enables you to clean under the gums as effectively as possible. Also, get toothbrushes with soft bristles. If your teeth start to show signs of sensitivity, ease up on your pressure and use very little or no toothpaste. You may have to even go back to your regular toothbrush for a while. Do not be as aggressive when you use your powered toothbrush the next time.

Are water irrigation devices useful

What about water irrigation devices? They are a great tool for the patient with deep periodontal pockets and if used correctly they can be very beneficial in assisting keeping the pockets cleaned. When cleaning out your perio pockets be careful to avoid turning the pressure to high, as you can damage the periodontal ligaments. For the majority of people they are acceptable to use if they are not being used as a substitute for brushing and flossing. They will not clean as effectively. It would be similar to washing your dirty car with only a power sprayer. It removes most of the dirt, but doesn't clean the car as well as washing it with a cloth and soapy water. The choice is up to you.

DECAY OR CAVITIES

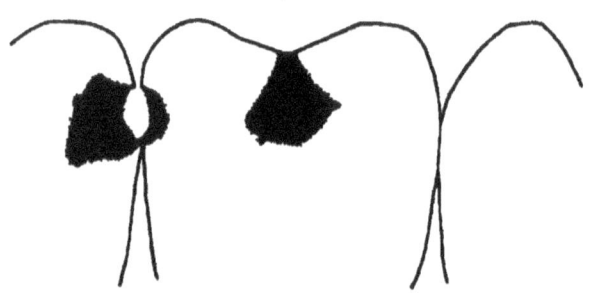

The decayed area of your tooth may look very small to you, but what you cannot see can be very large. Have your teeth checked by a dentist yearly.

One of the most widely spread diseases among humans is dental decay. It is also one of the easiest to prevent (refer to the sections on brushing and flossing).

Decay is caused by plaque being left on your teeth. Underneath the plaque, bacteria are trapped and combine with carbohydrates from your food. This ferments and produces acid, which is trapped and protected by the plaque. The acid then attacks the enamel on your teeth. This is known as decalcification and you may first notice it as an area on your teeth that looks chalky. If you begin taking care of it at this point you can still stop it. There are now products designed to help you remineralize that enamel that has been weakened.[5] If decay has entered into the enamel, but not into the dentin, it is known as incipient decay. This is what your dentist has the assistant notate to watch when you

---

[5] Example: MI Paste by GC America, Dental Products Report 2011-10.

have an exam. If you keep it clean you can slow it down and even stop it at that point. If not it will break through the enamel and become full blown decay. Once decay has broken through the enamel, it will spread through the dentin quickly. This is because dentin is not as hard as enamel. When left alone it can take months or years before it will reach the point where you will lose your tooth. This all depends on how well you take care of your teeth and how hard or soft your teeth are.

Decay will usually start between your teeth and on the top or biting surface of your back teeth. If you leave plaque on your teeth around the gum line, you'll also get decay started in that area as well. Decay can be misleading because while you may see a small hole on the surface of the tooth, below the surface the decay will mushroom or spread out. Once your enamel has decayed, it is gone and you cannot get it back. At best, you could get it restored by a good dentist. That tooth is now affected permanently. It doesn't have to get to this point however. Decay is easy to prevent when following correct brushing and flossing techniques.

TEMPORARY FILLINGS

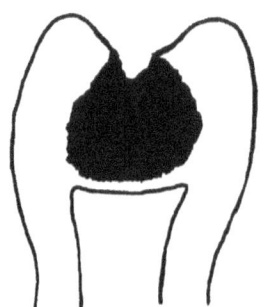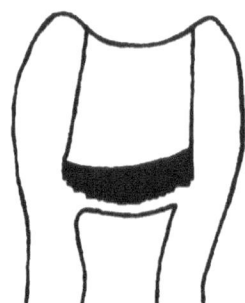

If you have large amounts of decay, talk with your dentist about the options before you begin treatment. If you take an interest and show you know something about what is going on, you are more likely to get the treatment you want. By removing the decay, followed by a base such as calcium hydroxide, then a temporary filling placed and left for about six months, many teeth can be saved from root canals or needing to be pulled (extracted).

There are times when your dentist will recommend a temporary filling. Let me help you understand what this is and why you would need it.

This type of temporary filling is not used as much as it could be, but it is an alternative you should be aware of. When your dentist is working on your teeth and removing decay, they may get very close to the nerve (pulp chamber). They may tell you that you now need a root canal or the tooth needs to be pulled (extracted).

However, all the decay does not necessarily need to be removed at your first dental appointment. If the dentist will stop short of exposing the nerve, they can use a base material such as calcium hydroxide or a light cured resin-modified calcium-silicate over the nerve/pulp and a temporary filling over that.[6] It is then left alone for up to 6 months. This treatment can sometimes save that tooth and you would not need a root canal or have it pulled (extracted). This is called an indirect pulp cap. If the pulp is exposed the same treatment is used, but it is then called a direct pulp cap.

The reason this works is the calcium hydroxide and the resin-modified calcium-silicate causes a secondary growth of dentin over the pulp/nerve. Many times this will grow thick enough in 6 months to allow the dentist to then remove all the decay and put in a permanent filling or crown if needed. This is a good option if conditions are right. Please understand that not all dentists believe these options work and they may not want to try them. Have them explain your options at this point and then decide what you want to do. Also understand that you do run some risk because you do not know how that tooth will react once you leave the dental office. You could have it abscess (read section on an abscess). If you elect to have this process used, request it in advance of the dentist working on you so they know you want to try it.

You must treat a temporary filling with extreme care. You cannot chew anything hard with it or you may cause too much trauma to the nerve or the temporary filling may break out. You must continue to brush and floss it, but be careful not to dislodge it. Your dentist can also take the tooth slightly out of occlusion so you don't bite as hard on it. There is a thought that the older you are, the less likely this method will be successful for you. If you are middle aged or older, you will not grow secondary dentin as fast, if at all. However, if you are in good health and want to try it then go for it. You may be successful. Be aware that there are risks with this procedure.

---

[6]   Example: TheraCal LC Protective Liner, BISCO Dental Products, wwwbisco.com

Sometimes temporary fillings are used to calm down a tooth that is very sensitive. Some temporary filling materials contain eugenol that has a sedative effect on your teeth. It can take some time, but it can help save your tooth and prevent more extensive work.

Sometimes temporary fillings are placed when many teeth are badly decayed. The dentist may remove all the decay on several teeth at the same visit knowing they will not have the time to fill them with permanent restorations. They do this to get the decay out and stop it from further destroying your teeth. Once they get all the decay out, they put the temporary fillings in and will place a permanent filling or what ever is required at a later date. The important thing is that you must return and have the work completed. Temporary fillings are just that, temporary. They are not meant to last for more than a few months.

Temporary fillings are also used when the dentist is not sure if the tooth will abscess or not. They place a temporary filling, perhaps give you antibiotics and then have you wait awhile for additional treatment. If the tooth survives, a filling is placed. If not, a root canal is done or the tooth is pulled.

Temporary fillings may also be in the form of a stainless steel, plastic or aluminum crown. This is placed over a tooth that is badly broken down or has been prepared for a crown. This type of temporary filling is designed to protect your tooth from breaking down. A word of caution about this type of temporary crown; they often have large overhangs which trap debris and bacteria. This can lead to gum problems, so be sure to brush and floss around them. *When you floss around this type of filling, pull your floss out not up or down.* Be sure to return to your dentist as soon as possible and have the temporary crown removed and replaced with a more permanent restoration or crown.

Each type of temporary filling has advantages for which it is designed; however, each can have a disadvantage as well. A temporary filling material designed to be used with a root canal tooth draws moisture from the tooth. It is not designed to be used on a vital (living) tooth. If it is used on a vital tooth, it will also draw moisture from that tooth and, in effect, cause it to become very sensitive and most likely die. Since you will not know the difference, have your dentist explain what type of temporary filling material is being used, they will give you one that they have used and are confident with its results. If you do not want an explanation, just ask for one that contains eugenol if your tooth is alive and you should be ok. You can smell the eugenol when it is placed into your tooth, it has a smell and taste of cloves. However it may not be your best option.

SILVER FILLINGS

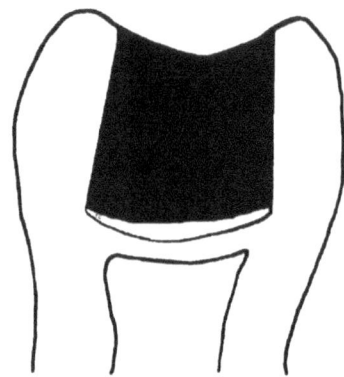

Silver is a common type of filling material. It is very strong and durable. It is one of the best filling materials we have available.

Silver fillings have been around for a long time and have improved over the years. Most people who have fillings will have some of this type. Silver fillings are also known as alloys, or amalgams. I will refer to them as alloys.

There are different types of alloys, each with its own properties. If you see one dentist, they may use one type and another dentist will use something different. It is unreasonable to expect the same result from both. Alloys are like cars. You have different qualities in each, and each one will perform differently based on those qualities. You have inexpensive alloys and better, more expensive alloys. It does not hurt to ask your dentist which type they are using and why. When speaking about fillings you must keep in mind that each filling is unique. There are variables associated with each tooth, which will not provide the exact same results each time.

When an alloy is placed into your tooth, the dentist who places it should place a base or insulator under the alloy. If the cavity had any depth at all, your tooth is going to be sensitive to hot and cold. This can continue for up to a year and maybe longer if there is no base or insulator. This is because the alloy is a conductor of temperature to the nerve of the tooth. There are different types of base materials, some are thin and flow easily and provide good results and some are thick and also provide good results. You have to trust your dentist regarding the type of base they select for your filling. However, always ask for some base, as a little protection is better than none.

If you have a tight contact between your teeth. You should expect the dentist to restore that same tight contact when they place a filling into your mouth. If your teeth have open contacts or wide spaces, don't expect the dentist to close the space. If the space is small, maybe they can. However, if the space is large and they fill it in, you run the risk of the filling breaking because you will have unsupported alloy.

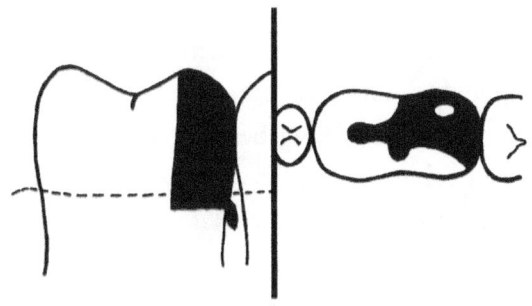

An amount of alloy formed below the margins of a tooth is called an overhang. It is very important that this be removed. If left in your mouth, it will trap debris and bacteria and be the starting place for decay and gum disease. A high spot on a filling (or a crown) will appear as a very shiny spot. It may be very small in size, but you must have it removed when you notice it. To neglect it could mean additional and very expensive dental work.

On occasion, when an alloy is placed, the dentist will leave an overhang which is a small outcrop of alloy located at the bottom of the filling; below the gum line. If this overhang is left on your tooth it will trap bacteria and acids that will attack your teeth and gums. There shouldn't be an overhang. The dentist should run floss between your teeth before they finish. If the floss catches, there is possibly an overhang. They should remove it right then. It will take additional time, but it is very important to your dental health to have it removed. You deserve to have it done correctly.

If an overhang is left you will not be able to properly clean under it and sometimes even between your teeth. This also results in developing gum disease, bone loss, and more cavities. This is why it is important to get the overhang removed before you leave the office. If you notice it after you leave the office, go back and have it removed as soon as you can. There should be no charge if that dentist is the one who did the filling. Whenever you have X-rays taken of your teeth, look at them yourself and have the dentist point out any overhangs or any other things that may be wrong with your teeth.

Be aware of any high spots

Another thing you should watch for with a new filling is something called a high spot. On new and sometimes even old fillings, you will feel your teeth hitting the filling before your other teeth come into contact with each other. It may also show up as a shiny spot. If you notice one, it means you are hitting that small spot before the rest of your teeth are coming into contact. If you have a shiny spot, return to your dentist as soon as possible and have it removed, do not delay. There are two reasons for having this done as quickly as possible. First, you don't want to risk breaking out the filling. Second, as you keep hitting this tooth you are causing trauma to the nerve. The tooth will only take a certain amount of trauma before it dies. If it dies, you may go through a lot of pain. You are also looking at a root canal, a crown, or needing that tooth pulled. This can possibly be avoided by having the high spot removed when it is noticed. It is painless to remove and can be done in a couple of minutes.

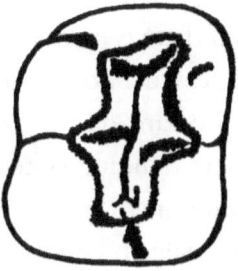 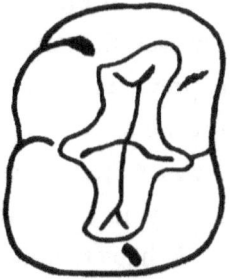

*The filling on the left has margins that have expanded and are
tarnished. These break off easier and will lead to more decay.
The filling on the right has been polished and the margins will not
expand much. This filling will last longer and not
break down as easily.*

Filling polished

Another thing to consider if you have alloys is to have them polished.
It is sometimes done on a subsequent visit, usually 1 to 4 weeks later.
The advantage in having your fillings polished is that they will last you
longer. If done correctly, they will be very smooth and shiny and look
like a gold crown or inlay, except they will be silver. Be sure when they
are polishing your fillings, they do not speed up the handpiece really
high and put a lot of pressure on the filling at the same time. This can
create a lot of friction and heat and could result in a dead nerve and
the need for a root canal and crown. I've had all of my fillings polished.
They wear and feel better and I want them to last as long as possible. I
do not like having them replaced.

Amalgam bonding

There has been a great improvement in recent years concerning alloys
called amalgam bonding.[7] It is a procedure that bonds alloys together
and bonds alloys to dentin and enamel. The advantage of this procedure

---

[7]   Example: All-Bond 2, BISCO Dental Products, wwwbisco.com

is that if you break off a piece of tooth or alloy, you don't always have to have the whole alloy removed and replaced if there is no decay present. With the previous method, every time you had an alloy replaced, you would lose some of your tooth structure. You can't do that too many times or you would be wearing crowns. The bonding system allows you to have your tooth repaired with minimum to no loss of tooth structure. Perhaps the biggest advantage of amalgam bonding is it can eliminate the leakage around the fillings that you now get. In some types of fillings, it will even strengthen the natural tooth structure. It also seals the inside of the tooth and cuts down on the sensitivity with little or no base added. This allows the dentist to place the maximum amount of alloy into the filling, reducing the chances that the filling will fracture. It can also eliminate the need to have pins put in your teeth to support and give retention to your fillings. All of the advantages of using amalgam bonding are not fully studied yet. It will do a lot of neat things for you

There has been a lot said about the use of mercury in dental alloys. There has been a big effort by some to educate people into thinking that mercury may be harmful to them and they must get their alloy fillings replaced with composites, ceramics or even crowns. One dentist I talked with on this subject said that dental alloys were still among the best restorative material we have at present, and the likelihood it will harm anyone is very slight. There are those who will have a genuine allergy to the mercury, but they will be very few. I don't profess to know the answers on this issue, but I think it is worth mentioning so you will be aware that the potential may be there if you have an allergy. If the potential is not there, there is no need to replace your fillings unless they need it for some other reason. This is a very good question to discuss with your dentist if you have concerns.

COMPOSITE RESTORATIONS

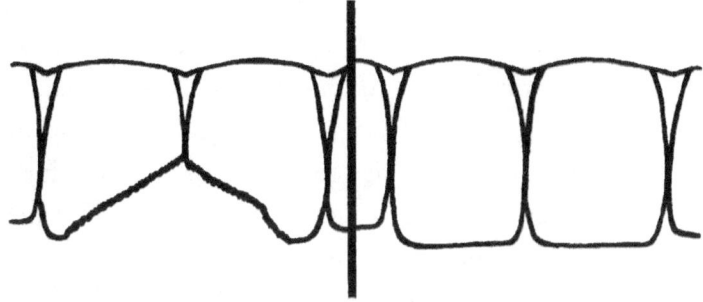

The loss of a portion of a front tooth as illustrated on the left is unsightly and possibly painful. Have the tooth fixed as soon as possible to prevent additional problems. By using a composite material, your dentist can restore the portion of tooth you have lost as illustrated on the right. Many times the color of your tooth can be matched so well it cannot be detected.

Composite restorations are the tooth colored filling material used on our front teeth, rather than using silver or gold. It has been a blessing to all of us who have lost a portion of our front teeth.

There are two common types of composites: self-cured and light-cured. The self-cured type comes as two pastes that are mixed together. After they are mixed, the dentist has 2 to 3 minutes to place it onto the patient's tooth before it becomes hard. After it hardens, the dentist will shape it and polish it. The light-cured type is a single paste that is placed onto the tooth and shaped. It then has an ultraviolet light placed on it that activates the material and makes it hard. A caution though, if you have the light used on your teeth, don't look directly at it. It has the potential to cause eye damage.

There are different sized particles in the composite materials which determine how hard they will be and how well they will polish. Your dentist should select the one that is appropriate for the type of restoration you need. You may ask your dentist why they have selected a certain type for you.

Acid etching and bonding is a technique used when a solution of phosphoric acid is used first on the teeth to etch them, and then a liquid resin is applied before the composite is placed. This bonds the composite to the enamel and dentin. This technique has the advantage that little, if any, of your healthy tooth structure has to be removed, as is done when mechanical retention is needed. Another advantage of bonding is that there is no margin between the natural tooth and the filling material. They are bonded or welded together. This bonding helps eliminate fillings falling out so easily.

This technique has the advantage of allowing other cosmetic applications to be done such as narrowing spaces between your teeth, covering surfaces that are broken, chipped, or worn, and covering badly stained teeth. I have had my teeth extended using this technique to replace enamel that I have worn off. The thing to remember with these types of restorations is that you cannot bite hard things like hard candy and ice. Doing so may break your restorations out, so be careful. The composite will also stain if you do not take good care of it. Things that will stain it the fastest are: tobacco, coffee, tea and certain types of juices. If you want to retain its nice appearance you'll have to take care of it.

There are many brands of composite on the market.[8] Some are better than others for one thing but not for other things. It is hard to get one which will do it all. Some brands come in many shades that the dentist can try to match with your teeth. Some come in only one shade. Don't be afraid to talk with your dentist to find out what you are receiving and why. Generally, the ones with several shades cost more.

---

8   Example: Ceram-X, Dentsply Caulk, wwwcaulk.com

However the dentist may have a fixed price for composites, so get what you want.

Watch your gum tissue around the teeth being worked on. If the dentist does not contour and polish the material right, you will have a food trap. This could be an overhang or just a rough filling. Test it with floss. If it catches, you have a problem. This can lead to gum infection and its associated problems. Catch it quickly and return to your dentist. If they put it in, they should correct it at no cost to you.

ABSCESS

One of the terms used in dentistry that puts fear and pain into the minds of patients is an abscess. How do you know you have an abscess? You'll have pain! There is almost always severe pain. It is intensified when you tap with something solid on the top of your tooth or try to eat. You may notice pus around your teeth and a foul taste and odor in your mouth.

There are two types of dental abscesses: periapical and periodontal. A periapical abscess will form at the end of a tooth (the apex). It will affect the bone and, if not treated right away, can destroy large portions of bone which supports the tooth. It has also affected the pulp or nerve of a tooth. It means the tooth has died, or in the process of dying.

The periodontal abscess affects the soft tissues around the teeth. This type will also result in the loss of soft tissue and, if not corrected, the loss of bone support. This type is treated by having your teeth cleaned by a dentist or hygienist and keeping them clean. You may be given antibiotics. This abscess may be caused by getting something wedged down deep between your teeth or under your gum tissue. Common causes can be pieces of toothpicks and popcorn hulls getting stuck. If you feel pain around your teeth try using your dental floss and see what you can remove. Be very careful in doing this. You usually cannot cure this condition on your own. If the pain persists, see your dentist as soon as possible because you will need help in getting this under control.

If you have a periapical abscess, you have 3 choices you can make. The first is to ignore it; however, it will not go away. If you ignore it, you are taking a gamble that you do not develop a very serious and even life threatening condition. *This can be very serious.* What it may also do is form a fistula or drainage hole through the bone and soft tissue. It will result in a release of pressure from the abscess and consequently, some relief from pain. It usually allows the pus from the infection to drain directly into your mouth. This depends on which tooth it is because it can also drain to other places such as your sinuses. You may be able to taste or smell it. Although the pain is relieved, it will continue to destroy bone and tissue until the source of the infection is removed. If allowed to continue for a long period of time, it increases the possibility that your overall health will be affected. *Remember as I mentioned before, it can become life threatening.* Do not ever think that it may go away or heal its self.

The second choice is to have a root canal done. This removes the nerves of the affected tooth and enables it to be saved. This will also eliminate the pain you were having. It is recommended that you be on antibiotics for several days before your root canal is started. This will eliminate or greatly lessen any pain you may have during the root canal procedure.

The third choice is to have the affected tooth pulled (extracted). In all cases, antibiotics are given to clear up the infection.

ROOT CANALS

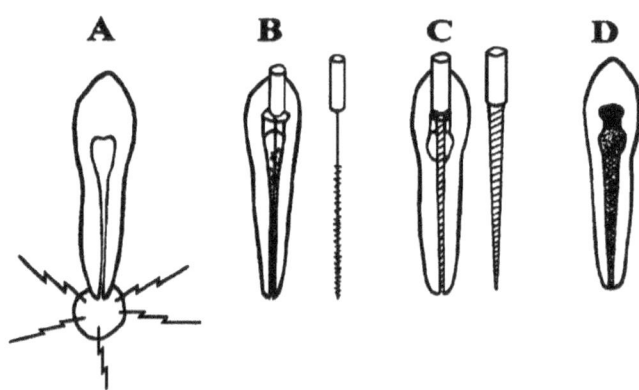

*The following steps are taken when a root canal is needed: (A.)
The tooth has abscessed. (B.) The nerve is removed from the
pulp chamber with an instrument called a broach. (C.) The pulp
chamber is cleaned out using a series of different sized files. (D.)
After the needed size is obtained, the pulp chamber is filled with a
soft material such as gutta-percha to seal off the chamber. A solid
filling is placed over the softer gutta-percha.*

I don't know of any dental procedure that brings fear to patients more than hearing they need a root canal. We all know someone who had the worst pain of their lives when a root canal was done. May I say that not all root canals are painful? Many are done without anesthetic and without pain. There are different reasons why a tooth would need a root canal. These reasons and the urgency with which the root canal must be done determine whether or not it will be painful.

I will give you a few possibilities of when a root canal may be necessary. Sometime during your life you may have been hit in the mouth. It could have been a fall, a car accident, a sporting accident, a fight with someone, almost any reason. The point is that you took a hard blow to your teeth. Depending on how hard the blow was and your general health, you could have problems right away or wait for years before you notice any effects. It usually begins with a change of color in your tooth. This can range from dark yellow or brown to dark gray or black. You may not have any discomfort. The change of color is an indication that the nerve in your tooth has died. If it has, you need to consider a root canal. This does not mean you need a root canal right away. You may go for years without any pain. What you may not know is that your tooth or teeth will become brittle as time goes on. This increases your possibility of a fracture on that tooth. All teeth with dead nerves will become brittle over time. One thing you can do is to have your dentist take your tooth, or as many teeth as necessary, out of occlusion so you are not biting as hard on them.

If you don't mind the changed color of your tooth or teeth, you can wait. If the color bothers you, then you need a root canal done before you have any other treatment such as a bleaching or crown. This is because you cannot change the color of the tooth by doing a vital (alive) bleaching. To bleach it, you must access the inside of the tooth. To do that you must clean out the pulp chamber and canal, or in other words do the root canal. Another option is to have a crown done. But if you have not had the root canal completed, the tooth can still abscess on you. Then the dentist would have to drill a hole through your crown to do the root canal. This can give you problems with your crown. Talk with your dentist, but I'm sure they will recommend having the root canal done before you have a crown if your tooth is in fact dead.

I've had three root canals and the dentist who did one of them had me wait a year before my crown was put on. This was to make sure my root canal was going to work because not all root canals are successful. I thought it was a good idea to wait. If the root canal didn't work, the tooth would need to be pulled and I would have wasted a lot of money on a crown. You can only wait like that if you have a full sized tooth to function with. If you only have part of a tooth, you would need a crown buildup and then the crown put on that. This should not be delayed because you need the space maintained so your other teeth do not drift.

Another reason making a root canal necessary is that you have allowed decay to enter the pulp chamber. This can be prevented by seeing your dentist regularly and having your teeth X-rayed. If you haven't been to your dentist, you may notice it yourself if you have a constant pain that never goes away or if you can see a lot of decay in your tooth. There are countless ways for decay to enter the pulp. Once this happens and if it is extensive enough you have two choices: pull the tooth or get a root canal. If you do nothing the tooth will decay and break apart, most likely abscessing and destroying bone and tissue around it. In short, it will give you a lot of pain and misery until you have it pulled.

When you have an accident and have your tooth broken at a level that involves the pulp chamber, the two choices mentioned above are your only options. In this situation, you usually can't put your choices off to a later date.

Another cause of trauma, though less common, that can result in the need for a root canal is a high spot on your new fillings or crowns. You can kill the nerve in one of the involved teeth and not know you are doing it. This is caused by the constant pounding it goes through when you eat or close your mouth. It is very important to have the high spot removed when you notice it so you can avoid killing the nerve. This has happened to several friends of mine and to me. Believe me it was very painful until the antibiotics took affect and then I was able to have the root canals done.

Not all of these situations will result in painful root canals. For the tooth that has died and changed color, there is usually no pain at all. For the others, your dentist will numb up your tooth enough so you should not have any pain either. The only exception is a tooth that has abscessed and needs a root canal to be done right away. Understand that it is hard to get an abscessed tooth completely numb. If your dentist can give you some antibiotics for a few days, preferably 4 to 7, your abscess should go away enough so they can then get your tooth completely numb. This will allow you to have a relatively painless root canal. A word of caution, many patients after receiving their antibiotics and having the pain go away in a few days, think they can now get by without the root canal. *This is a bad idea!* The pain will come back, and continue doing so, until you have the root canal done. This is one of the reasons the dentist will begin a root canal on an abscessed tooth when you first see them. It is more painful but it does get the root canal started. If you can commit to returning in a few days, it is far less painful to get the antibiotics and then come back to start the root canal.

There may also be instances when you need a root canal and do not know it. This is because you can have a tooth with an abscess that is not giving you pain. There are usually two reasons for this. The first is that you may have decay or some other reason that there is an opening into the pulp chamber of a tooth. This will allow the pus to drain through the pulp chamber into your mouth. The second reason is that the tooth can form what is called a fistula. This is a small canal or opening between the abscess and usually the soft tissue of the mouth. However it can also go into other areas such as your sinuses. It goes through the bone and soft tissue and can form a small bump on the side of your gum tissue. This can enlarge until it is ruptured and drains into your mouth. Either way, because the pus can drain you do not have the pain you would otherwise have. However, you do have the pus draining into your mouth which you usually swallow. Over a period of time this can affect your overall health and the way you feel. If these openings get plugged up, you will get pressure to build up and have the pain associated with an abscess. Keep a good watch on any tooth you suspect of having an abscess and get it checked by your dentist as soon as possible. *An abscess can become life threatening if untreated.*

How is a root canal done

When you get a root canal, the root canal will be cleaned out with sterile instruments called broaches and files. Many dentists now use ultrasonic files that clean out the canal much faster. The cleaning out of the canals may take several appointments depending on the condition and the teeth involved. It is then filled with a filling material such as gutta-percha which is a soft material that can be condensed into the cleaned canal and seal the canal off.

My last word on root canals is to remember that your teeth will become brittle after you have one. You will need a crown. Also, have your tooth or teeth checked to see if you have a good bone level of support around your teeth. If you don't have the bone support, don't even consider the root canal because you won't be able to keep the tooth anyway. Remember that as much as dentist try, not every root canal is successful. Some do fail and then more treatment is needed or the tooth has to be pulled. If you suspect that your tooth will be very difficult to be worked on, you may want to consider seeing an Endodontist who is specialized in doing difficult root canals. I highly recommend them after having my own tooth abscess on me and needing a difficult root canal done.

TEETH WHITENERS AND BLEACHING

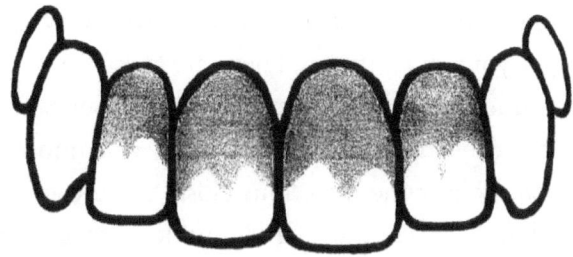

Most everyone wants white, beautiful teeth and there are many products that will help you have them. Many you can apply yourself and many need to be applied by your dentist. If you do not achieve the results you want, see your dentist and do not give up.

Both of these terms have the same effect (to make your teeth whiter and more attractive) so I will discuss them together.

I have performed a lot of bleaching procedures and I've seen some excellent results. I recommend when you have your teeth bleached, you do it in a dental office and under controlled conditions. The dentist may use a rubber dam on your teeth that will isolate the teeth and protect your gums and other soft tissues.

Most of the bleaching procedures I did were done using a mixture which was activated with heat. This mixture worked on vital (alive) and non-vital (dead) teeth. For vital teeth, the mixture was placed on the teeth and then heat was applied either with a hot instrument or a light which generated heat. This type of treatment usually took several visits. For non-vital teeth (a tooth with a root canal) there is a technique called a walking bleach. The mixture is placed into the pulp chamber of a non-vital tooth and left for about 7 days. When you return to the dentist the mixture is removed and if the desired results are met a filling is placed in the tooth. If the results are not what you want, they will do it again. We bleached the tooth to a point that was just slightly lighter (whiter) than the adjacent teeth because it would darken up a little after we were finished.

There has been controversy about self-applied tooth whiteners for years. Problems associated with this option were that not only were the results very temporary, but you could end up with very sensitive teeth and damage to your gum tissue. There are many new self applying whitening products on the market that offer outstanding results. However, because I have not had experience with most of them let me caution you. Follow the directions closely! You can easily damage your teeth and gums if you don't. If you notice any pain or unwanted change in the condition of your teeth or gums, stop using the product. Many of our patients who used the self applied whiteners, experienced increased sensitivity to their teeth. If your teeth start to get sensitive, stop using the product. Whiter teeth that are sensitive and painful are of no advantage. My recommendation is to have a dentist give you the whitening treatment. They know what they are doing and they have access to products you don't. They can also closely follow procedures while protecting your teeth and gums.

Many of us do not have teeth that are the color we want them to be. We all want white teeth. However, teeth usually vary in shade from light yellow to dark brown or gray. You may not believe me, but many people do not have naturally white teeth. Most of us have a slight discoloration in our teeth. It is usually not noticeable unless the color of our teeth is very dark.

Causes for discoloration

There are several causes for the discoloration. It could be caused by use of the antibiotics of the tetracycline group. If these antibiotics are administered between the second trimesters of pregnancy to the approximate age of 8, it can result in permanent discoloration of the teeth. This color can range from a light yellow or gray to a dark gray.

Another common cause is a stain known as fluorosis. Fluorosis occurs when excessive amounts of fluoride are ingested (taken internally), during the same period of time as mentioned above. This will usually happen in areas where the water is naturally too high in fluoride content. The US specifies the optimal level of fluoride to range from 0.7 to 1.2 mg/L (milligrams per liter, equivalent to parts per million), depending on the average daily air temperature.[9] The severity of the stain, which can range from minor to severe brown, will depend on how much fluoride was actually ingested.

Other types of stain are caused by what we put into our mouths. Things such as tobacco, coffee, tea and some types of foods and juices will stain our teeth. Most of these stains can be removed by a hygienist or by having your teeth bleached. After you have the stains removed, you will get them back unless you give up whatever it was that caused the stains. Keeping your teeth clean is the best way to reduce the amount of stain you get.

In the first two instances above, the ingestion of antibiotics and too much fluoride, the best treatment is to have the teeth bleached by a dentist, or have the teeth covered with a veneer. These forms of treatment are very good, but keep in mind that they will possibly need follow-up. The bleaching will last a long time, but usually not forever and the veneers could fall off or break and need replacement. For those who want the veneers there are new bonding materials that could keep the veneers on for many years, if not for your lifetime, depending how

---

[9]   Wikipedia, en.wikipedia.org/wiki/Water_fluoridation

you take care of them. A full crown is the closest form of permanent treatment, but you may be cutting down a healthy tooth and ending up with other problems. A full crown should be considered only as a last option.

TOOTH ABRASION AND EROSION

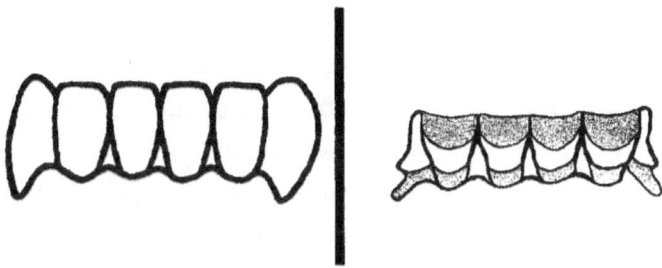

The teeth on the left represent normal teeth. The teeth on the right represent teeth that have large areas missing due to erosion or abrasion. Teeth in this condition may not have any pain, however as the erosion nears the pulp chamber you increase your chances of having pain and having the teeth fracture.

If you look at your teeth and notice a groove cut into your teeth along the gum line or your teeth are showing a great deal of wear on the top and front side you have abrasions or erosion.

This condition is caused by a combination of things. Any toothpaste that is abrasive will tend to wear down the teeth. Using a hard toothbrush can also be a big contributor. If you are doing both of these things and brushing incorrectly, you're almost guaranteed to have this problem.

To prevent this type of abrasion use gentle non-abrasive toothpaste in a small amount and a soft or extra soft toothbrush. When brushing, angle your toothbrush toward the gums and gently message your teeth and gums.

Another cause for this condition is eating too many foods or drinks with high acid content, such as sodas and citrus fruits. Some people who are bulimic and vomit frequently may also have this problem. The erosion of the teeth is one of the first indicators of a person who is bulimic but is trying to hide it. It affects the teeth and cannot be hidden.

If your gums have receded, you may get grooves on the root portion of the tooth. They will wear down faster than the crown of the tooth because the roots are softer than the enamel that covers the crown. If the erosion is extensive enough, the treatment is to have a filling placed in that area. In the past this type of problem would not always be filled because you had to remove good tooth structure in order to place the filling. With the newer bonding techniques, your dentist can bond a filling over the eroded area and not have to remove any or very little of your tooth structure. You must be aware that this type of restoration may not last if you do not watch how you eat and take care of your teeth.

You may experience sensitivity with this condition even before you notice the erosion. That is because you have irritated the gums so much they have receded and exposed the root of the tooth. If this happens quickly, before the teeth adjust, you will notice a lot of sensitivity to hot and cold. When you breathe in air or touch this area you will have a sharp pain that goes away after a while.

Treatment for this type of sensitivity is to use desensitizing toothpaste, along with the proper care mentioned earlier. You can also see your dentist who can give you a treatment using a strong fluoride solution, but this is usually a temporary thing. A recent form of treatment, which shows good indications of being longer lasting, is to have the dentist cover the sensitive area with the bonding liquid only, using no composite. Early indications for this type of treatment are very promising.

Grinding your teeth

Teeth grinders not only wear down their teeth, but they also put a great deal of pressure on the TMJ (Temporomandibular Joint). This can cause them to have severe pain in the joint area and even lead to severe headaches. For those who grind their teeth it is not as easy to correct. Teeth grinding can be the result of several things, but it is felt that stress is the most common cause. During the day a person can consciously think about it and control it to an extent, but during the night it is a different situation. Most people grind their teeth the hardest while they are asleep. It can be a noisy habit and an irritation to those around them. If you have this problem, may I suggest you see your dentist as soon as possible? Your dentist will give you some ideas to help prevent your grinding problem, but they will also suggest that you consider using a device called a night guard (mouth guard). Impressions are taken of your teeth and the night guard is made specifically for your mouth. Your dentist will make any adjustments necessary so that it will fit as comfortable as you can get wearing something in your mouth. The night guard will be made of acrylic and inserted over your teeth each night before you go to sleep. You will likely still grind your teeth, but you will be grinding on the night guard and not your teeth. This will prevent the abrasion and wearing down of your teeth. It will often reduce the pain you may be getting in the TMJ area as well. Some people have even been able to eliminate teeth grinding as a problem after using a night guard, so you may want to consider trying one.

BLEEDING GUMS

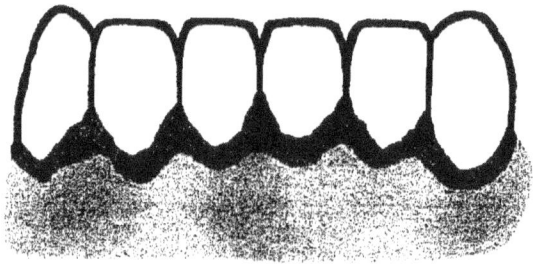

The way bleeding gums are started: (A.) Plaque forms a hard material called tartar. This tartar irritates the gum tissues and they become infected and bleed. (B.) The tartar has increased in size and the bone may recede away. The gum tissue bleeds very easily and becomes swollen.

Bleeding gums is a very prevalent disease and it can run from slight to severe. It usually is caused by dental plaque. I say usually because there are many different factors which can cause bleeding gums including stress, poor nutrition and medical conditions such as diabetes or taking blood thinners. If you have swollen and bleeding gums, try the things I'm suggesting for a couple of weeks. If your gums do not heal and stop bleeding or at least show improvement, see your dentist or physician for their evaluation. If you have tartar on your teeth, you should see a dentist or hygienist and have it removed. It will act as a trap until it is removed.

The best time to get control of bleeding gums is when you first notice it. This will usually be when you are brushing your teeth. The reason they are bleeding is because you are developing a gum infection called gingivitis. It is nothing to be alarmed at in the beginning stages.

It can be controlled or eliminated and you can often do it yourself. If your bleeding problem is isolated to only a few areas, find these areas and be conscientious about keeping them clean. You will not usually develop a gum infection in a mouth that is kept clean.

To clear up this problem, start by better brushing and flossing. Are you surprised? Don't be. Those of you who brush and floss regularly are usually never bothered with this problem. Refer to the sections on brushing and flossing to see how you can improve on your technique. Don't be surprised when you start flossing if your gums become tender and bleed a little for a few days. This is a common reaction but you must not give up! After a couple of weeks, you will be happy to see your bleeding problem is going away, if not completely eliminated.

Another thing you can do is to use a mouth rinse. There are commercial rinses that may help you or your dentist can give you a prescription for one, if you have enough of a problem.[10] However, let me save you some money. One of the best rinses is warm salt water. It doesn't have all the flavoring, but it is effective. Just don't make it so salty you get sick using it. Use it about three times during the day.

If gingivitis is left alone because it hurts, it will get worse. As it gets worse it progresses to periodontitis. This means it has gone from being a gum problem to one involving the periodontal ligaments and the bone that supports the teeth. You are now in a situation that requires the help of a dentist. The sooner you see a dentist, the less bone destruction you will have. Remember, it will still be a condition which depends on you to clear it up. The dentist and hygienist will help you, but you have the biggest responsibility. The key is to brush and floss effectively and regularly.

---

[10] Example: PerioMed Oral Rinse Concentrate, 3M ESPE, www.3mespe. com

GUM DISEASE
(PERIODONTAL DISEASE)

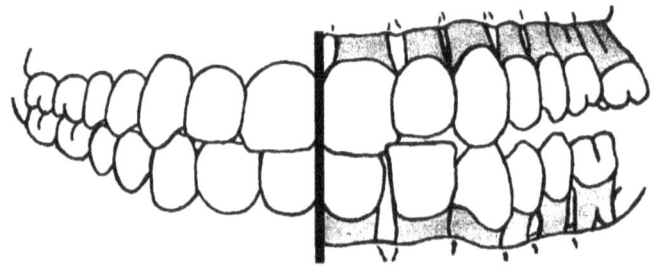

This is a comparison of a healthy mouth on the left and one with advanced gum disease (periodontal disease) on the right. The receding gums are usually a result of neglect. Plaque left on the teeth form a hard material called tartar. This tartar irritates the gum tissue and the gums recede. As the gums recede, the bone underneath will also recede. The roots are exposed and the teeth may become loose and possibly drift out of position. A very foul odor is usually present. Proper cleaning will help you avoid this condition and keep your teeth and gums healthy.

Many articles have been written about gum disease, yet most people know nothing about it. Almost every person has been affected to some degree with gum disease (hereafter called perio). There are many causes for perio disease. Some of these you have limited control over such as an injury, puberty, pregnancy, mouth breathing and medications. There are also other reasons, so check with your dentist if you suspect it could be one of these. However, the major cause of perio disease is the neglect of people to keep their teeth free of plaque and tartar.

If your gums are bleeding when you brush your teeth you may have gingivitis, which is perio in a mild stage. At this stage it can easily be treated and cured. All you may have to do is start brushing and flossing correctly. If you do not have a lot of tartar on your teeth, the bleeding should stop within a few weeks. If it doesn't stop, see your dentist right away for an exam. It will likely be treatable with a cleaning by a hygienist.

If you do not treat the bleeding problem, it may get worse. Many people will slack off on their brushing and flossing because it hurts. *Do not do that*! If anything, increase the amount of care given to your gums. Instead of healing your problem, slacking off on home care will make your problem worse. I'm not trying to scare you, but if totally neglected, you risk developing moderate to severe periodontal disease and perhaps the condition called ANUG (Acute Necrotizing Ulcerative Gingivitis). Some of you know this condition by its old name "trench mouth." This is a painful and destructive infection of the gums. It is also a condition which affects many young adults that are run down or under a lot of stress. Like advanced perio disease, this condition causes you to give off a foul odor from your mouth.

To treat ANUG, you will need an appointment with your dentist or hygienist for a gross debridement, or the removal of most of your plaque and tartar. This will usually be done with the assistance of an anesthetic because your gums at this stage are very painful. You will be given home cleaning instructions, nutrition counseling, rest instructions, and possibly an antibiotic.[11] It will be necessary to see your dentist again for a more thorough cleaning when your mouth can handle it better. Don't miss that appointment!

Perio will creep up on you

One of the bad things about perio is that it is a slow and painless disease in most cases. It can take years of neglect before you will notice any destruction of the bone that supports your teeth. Most of us will fit into this category. It is surprising to see patients who have little or no

---

[11]   Including sufficient amounts of Vitamins C, D and Calcium.

decay, or other dental problems, and yet they lose their teeth because of bone loss. The real tragedy is they didn't know it until it is sometimes too late. Many are in disbelief or even outraged when they find out they may lose their teeth. You may have no visible symptoms, no bleeding gums and no pain. Most but not all will be near 40 years of age before they find out they have perio disease. They have spent a lifetime taking care of their teeth to prevent decay because that's all they were taught. They should have been taking more care of their gums and supporting bone. When doing this correctly, they also prevent decay.

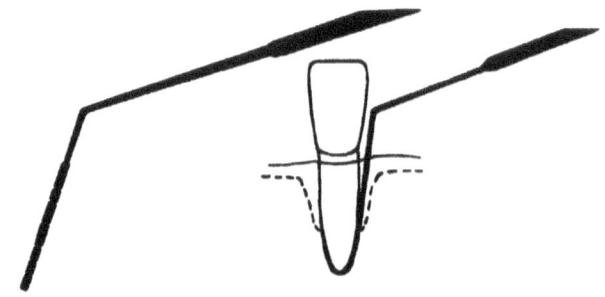

Your dentist can check the amount of bone loss around your teeth by using a perio probe. If the probe goes to any depth over 3 mm you have periodontal disease.

The way to find out if you have perio is to request your dentist look at your bitewing X-rays for decay and bone loss. Have them show you where your bone level is and explain what you can expect. Also have them check with a periodontal (perio) probe around all your teeth. The perio probe is marked with millimeter gradations from 1 to 10 mm, and is carefully inserted between the tooth and gum tissue. Those teeth that are not X-rayed will be checked in this way. Do this each year.

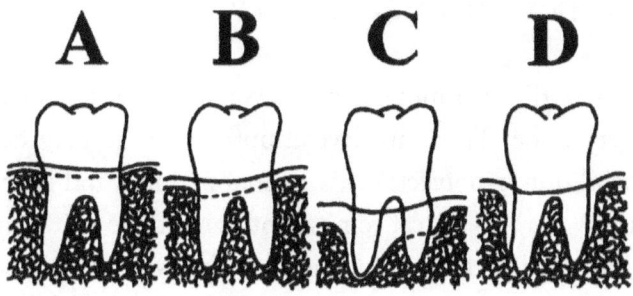

This illustrates the degrees of bone loss. (A) Normal bone. (B) Moderate bone loss, but little loss of gum tissue. (C) Severe bone loss and gum loss. The area between the roots of the tooth may also be exposed. (D) You can also have a deep perio pocket and not loose all the surrounding bone.

The periodontist I worked with considered any bone loss over 3 mm in depth to be perio disease. If you have perio disease there are several ways of treating it, depending on the severity of the disease. If not too involved, you may have it corrected with a teeth scaling and curettage. That is the cleaning away of the tartar and dead tissue from around your teeth. If it is more involved, you may have a perio pocket (a defect down the side of the tooth involving the destruction of the supporting bone). This condition may need a root planing. The tooth is first cleaned of all tarter with hand instruments and an ultra sonic scaler. The roots of the tooth are then scraped clean and smooth with hand instruments. It may be slightly contoured to remove the dead tissue in the periodontal pocket. This procedure is done with the aid of an anesthetic. This should leave the roots clean and smooth for the growth of secondary cementum and reattachment of the periodontal tissues in some cases.

Types of periodontal surgery

If your perio condition is more involved, you may need to look at having perio surgery done. There are several options for surgery depending on your condition: gingivectomy, a periodontal flap and laser surgery. Gingivectomy is the surgical removal of part of the soft tissue (your gums). This could include reducing the soft tissue over a pocket and extensive root planing after the walls of the pocket have been cleaned of diseased tissue. Those people who have gum tissue that has grown over their teeth because of medications will benefit from this type of perio surgery.

The perio flap is a more extensive type of perio treatment. The gum tissue is laid open so the entire tooth, perio pockets and infected bone are all exposed. The teeth are root planed, the pocket is cleaned out and all dead tissue and affected bone are removed. The bone is recontoured and all pointed areas removed. The infected gum tissue is removed. After all this is done, the gum tissue is then sutured (stitched) in place over the bone and a surgical dressing is placed to protect the surgery site. This is left on for about 5-7 days and then the sutures and dressing are removed.

The laser treatment is the newest development in periodontal care.[12] It enables your dentist to remove the diseased bone and tissue in a much less traumatic way. By using a laser, only the diseased tissue is removed along with the tarter. The procedure is much shorter in time, less painful and the healing time is about half that of the other methods. If you need this level of treatment, I would strongly recommend you check out the options and benefits of having the laser treatment done.

These sound like very painful procedures, but they really are not. Years ago, the periodontist I worked with preferred the perio flap method of treatment because it was the most thorough. However if I ever needed perio surgery, I'd now have the laser procedure done if it

---

[12]   Example: TLC for gums Therapeutic Laser care, www.TLC4Gums.com

were available. I'd want to make sure mine is completely taken care of with the least amount of trauma and the shortest healing time.

If you are ever in a position to have perio surgery, remember that if you have the surgery done, but do not take proper care of your teeth and gums, you'll soon be back in the same situation only it will be worse this time. I cannot emphasize enough that you must develop a habit of good, proper home care and follow-up with your dentist. Otherwise, don't waste your time and money to go through all that discomfort. Instead, hang in there as long as you want and then get your teeth pulled and get dentures. However, remember that proper home care is just thorough brushing and flossing on a daily basis.

At what point have you lost too much bone

People have asked me at which point have they lost too much bone support to consider perio surgery. This will vary with each person and with the type of home care you give your teeth. The rule of thumb is that if you have less than 1/2 to 1/3 of your bone support left, it is risky to consider. However, I have seen people maintain teeth in that situation for long periods of time, so anything is possible. But discuss with your dentist your options and potential outcomes before you make any decisions to have surgery.

You may have perio disease in some areas of your mouth and not in others, so you are not necessarily looking at having your whole mouth treated. Have your dentist give you a treatment plan and explain all that needs to be done and the areas to be treated.

If you have AIDS

For those who have AIDS: often AIDS is diagnosed because of gum disease that does not readily heal after you and your dentist have faithfully done everything you should. Your gum disease may be no different than those without AIDS, but the condition causes perio disease to manifest more severely and takes longer to heal. You must become very dedicated about proper home care. If you suspect you have been exposed to AIDS, have yourself tested.

My last comment on perio disease is that with very few exceptions, it can be prevented if you start taking proper care of your teeth, dental appliances and gums early enough. There is usually no need for anyone to lose their teeth because of bone loss.

BABY BOTTLE SYNDROME

One of the hardest things to see in any dental office is when a parent brings in their baby or toddler with baby bottle syndrome or nursing bottle mouth. This is rampant dental decay of the infant's teeth. Sometimes there are no crowns left on the teeth. It most often results when the infant is given a bottle containing a sweetened liquid very frequently. It especially is destructive when either milk or a sweetened liquid is given just before they go to sleep. The sugar in the liquid mixes with the bacteria in the dental plaque and forms the acid that causes the decay. When milk is given before going to sleep, lactic acid is produced which stays on the infant's teeth throughout the night and it continually attacks the teeth to destroy the enamel. You don't have as much of a problem when the child is awake because saliva will help carry the liquid away from the teeth.

May I suggest that if your child must have a bottle when they go to sleep, it is best to give them one that contains only water. Juices can have the same effect as milk or sweetened liquids. If your child needs something to suck on to go to sleep then you may want to consider using a pacifier. Make sure the pacifier is clean and do not put any type of sweetener on it.

If you are wondering at which age to start brushing your child's teeth to help prevent this condition, start before the first tooth erupts. Get them used to having you touch their gums. When the first tooth erupts, start brushing it with some form of a baby toothbrush or wipe with *no toothpaste*, or a very small amount of baby toothpaste which does not contain fluoride. Brush all the teeth thoroughly at least once a day, preferably in the evening before putting them to bed for the night.

If your child has started to show any signs of decay in their teeth, take them to a dentist as soon as possible. The dentist can remove the decay if not to extensive and put fillings in. They can also give you guidance on how to prevent more decay in the future. If your child has extensive decay, may I recommend that you take them to a pediatric dentist or pedodontist that is specifically trained to treat this condition in children.

CARING FOR YOUR CHILDREN'S TEETH

This area of dentistry could be a complete book all by itself. I will try to give you a few good ideas which will help you take better care of your children's teeth. You can start by getting your young children used to having you stick your finger into their mouth. Please wash your hands first. Gently massage your child's gum tissue before the first teeth are visible. After the teeth appear, gently brush them daily with a baby toothbrush or wipe. If you feel you must use toothpaste, please use toothpaste that is made especially for babies which does not contain fluoride. Do not let them get use to swallowing the toothpaste. In fact, you do not need to use any toothpaste at all because it is the toothbrush and not the toothpaste that will clean the teeth. As soon as they will let you, begin to floss their teeth. If they don't like it, back off until they are older and try again. A floss aid works well with children. Have them watch you, so that brushing and flossing is an acceptable practice to them. *Your example will be the key.*

When children are approximately age 2 to 3, have them visit a dentist for the first time. It is always best to take them before they develop decay or other dental problems. The first visit can be for a simple cleaning and fluoride treatment and perhaps a sealing if indicated. These are painless procedures and it gives the child a positive experience with the dentist so that they do not fear them. Often most of this will be done by the dentist's staff, with the dentist usually doing the exam. By getting them familiar with seeing the dentist, they become a friend and are happy to see them. They will not develop the fear which many of us have. Their first words to the dentist will not be "I hate you".

Something to be avoided

Things you should avoid: please don't ever threaten your child with going to the dentist or getting a shot in the mouth. They will instantly be afraid and never trust them, no matter how good the dentist and their staff are. They will fear going to the dentist throughout their lives just like many of you do now. They will not get problems taken care of early and will end up having the more extensive treatment done. They will often end up wearing dentures. This can all be avoided by how you introduce them to the dentist. It is up to you!

If your dentist determines that the child does need to have a filling or other treatment, don't be alarmed and don't show the fear you may have in your facial expressions. It is best if you don't say anything. Your child will pick up on your attitude instantly. Just let the dentist and their staff handle it. Techniques and dental materials have improved so much over the years that your child will most likely feel no pain and not have any problem at all. My granddaughter at age 5 was excited to show me the stars (fillings) her dentist put in her teeth. What a neat dentist she had that helped her have a good experience.

I suggest that if you have young children and especially if they have special needs that you take them to a pediatric dentist or pedodontist if one is available. They and their staff have very extensive training and experience which will make a big difference to your child no matter what their age is.

CROWNS

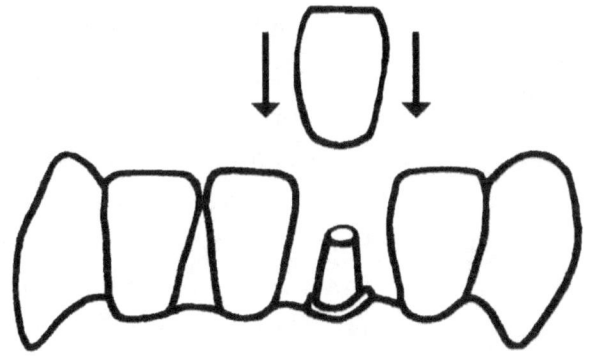

A tooth must be filed down for a crown to be made. Consider very carefully having good healthy teeth filed down as it lasts a lifetime.

Crowns are used to cover teeth that are discolored, broken, misshaped, have had root canals and are badly broken down because of decay. You may have one or all of your teeth crowned.

Before the introduction of bonding materials, it was not uncommon for your dentist to recommend you having a crown made whenever you have lost a cusp (off your back teeth) or a large portion of your front teeth. Because of the bonding materials available for alloys and composites, you can have your teeth repaired very well and for much less. If you have lost a major portion of your tooth however, you may want to consider having a crown made. A crown is stronger and has less chance of breaking than a restoration.

There are differences between dentists in preparing a tooth for a crown. Some will push the gum tissue back out of the way and prepare the tooth. Because the tissue is numb, you won't feel it and it heals quickly. Some cut the tissue out with the dental burs as they file the tooth down. This will leave the tissue very sore and it can take weeks to heal. I've had them done both ways and I prefer the first method. Ask your dentist before you have a crown done and take the method you prefer.

Crowns are made of gold, ceramic, gold/ceramic combination, nonprecious metals and nonprecious metals/ceramic combination. There is always a debate over which is best. You may want to have your dentist explain the differences between them in relation to where your tooth is located before you make a decision.

If you are going to have a crown on a front tooth, don't expect it to perfectly match the shade of your other teeth. It is hard to match what nature has given you by looking at a tooth shade guide and picking one to match yours. This is especially true if your teeth are shaded any shade other than perfectly white. The dentist will do their best to get a match as close as possible. You have a big advantage if your dentist does their own lab work, or if they have a lab technician come and take the shade themselves. Most dentists send their lab work to private labs and that lab can only go by what is written down on the lab prescription form. With your front teeth, the shade difference is not so noticeable when several teeth are crowned at the same time. This depends on the condition of the other teeth, the cost and how much it is worth to you.

After your crown is inserted, you should be able to use floss without catching the floss on the margins of the crown. If you catch the margins, you may have an overhang. Return to your dentist and have the margins adjusted. The margins that catch floss will also trap bacteria and debris. This will increase the possibility of getting decay under your crown. If you do not want to return to your dentist, be sure you floss and brush under the overhang. If you keep it clean, you lessen the possibility of getting decay. However, you really should return to your dentist and have the overhang removed. You paid to have your tooth fixed correctly, so get it done correctly.

Something for you to consider when having your crown cemented: talk with your dentist about having your crown bonded on instead of using regular cement. Studies indicate that it has the effect of eliminating the space along the margins, plus it should not wash out like regular cements do, thereby decreasing the possibility of decay. It also is reported to hold better and longer. It is more expensive though, and every dentist may not be using it. If you want it done, talk with your dentist before they begin.

Cautions

A few words of caution though before you consider having a crown made, know the periodontal condition of your tooth. If your tooth is not likely to last long or needs other extensive treatment, you may want to reconsider the investment. When the dentist is preparing your teeth, make sure they use a water spray to keep the tooth cooled down and that they do not grind off the tooth structure too fast. You may need to just trust your dentist to do this correctly. The reason I mention this is if a tooth is traumatized too much during this process, you can expect to come back and have a root canal done. That does not mean you still won't end up needing a root canal. Having a crown made may be too much trauma for the tooth, but you can lessen the possibility. This is a good question to discuss with your dentist before treatment is started.

If you get your crown inserted and leave the dental office then notice you hit the crown high (hit it before you hit your other teeth), return immediately or as soon as you can, and have the crown adjusted. If you continue to bite on this high spot, you risk killing the nerve because of the trauma you are creating on that tooth. It does not take long to do this damage; a few days could do it. If you kill the nerve, you are looking at a root canal or having the tooth pulled. That is a lot of additional expense and pain that you can possibly avoid. It will only take a couple of minutes to adjust the crown, and there should be no additional cost.

While I'm talking about crowns, let me mention temporary crowns. They are primarily used as an interim protection device while your teeth are being worked on. They are not designed to last for years, although some do. They are usually made of plastic, stainless steel or aluminum. They are adapted chairside by a dentist or an assistant and then cemented in place. The big problem with these is they often have open margins, large overhangs, and break or wear out easily. They can give you long lasting problems if they are left for long periods of time. You must keep the area around them clean. When flossing, do not pull your floss up and down to get it out. Release one end and pull it out. Do not chew on them, if possible. However, if you have to, avoid anything hard. If they break or come loose, get them replaced right away. See your dentist and have them replaced with something permanent as soon as you can.

BRIDGES

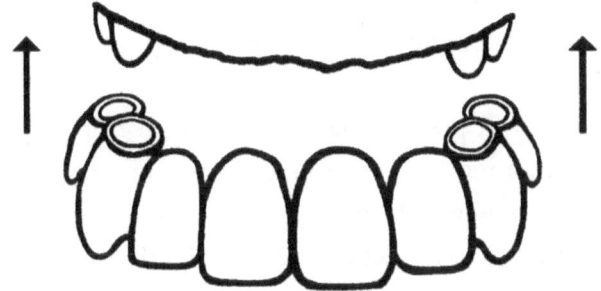

This illustrates an eight-unit bridge. There are two abutment teeth at each end and this will give you much more stability.

A bridge in a person's mouth is similar to a bridge we have all crossed over. It is anchored at each end and has a span in-between. The space in-between is filled with something resembling your natural teeth, both in appearance and function.

If you need a bridge, have the health of the anchor teeth evaluated before having it made. If they are involved with extensive bone loss, you may want more teeth pulled (extracted) before you get the bridge. Talk with your dentist and have them show you on your X-rays, where your current bone level is. Decide after you have an estimate of how long they can be expected to last. Be careful of using any teeth that are periodontally involved. They usually do not last without having extensive periodontal treatment. I would also be careful when considering using a bridge to stabilize teeth that have periodontal involvement. They usually are not successful unless you have total dedication to good oral hygiene.

Is a bridge necessary

Is a bridge necessary? That depends on the location of the missing teeth. As a rule, bridges serve several important functions. They help keep the teeth aligned in the mouth. The teeth will tend to drift forward into the empty space where the missing teeth were located. This can cause malocclusion problems. Your teeth will not bite the way they did before you lost the other teeth. Your appearance can be changed by this shifting as well, especially if the tooth is missing from the front of your mouth.

The bridge will prevent the opposing teeth from super erupting. In other words, a tooth will continue to grow and fill in the space on the opposing arch where the missing teeth were located. It will become longer than the adjacent teeth. This is unsightly and can cause other problems if left uncorrected. This is why dentists will advise you to replace any missing teeth with some form of false teeth as soon as possible.

You should consider waiting from 3 to 5 weeks after a tooth is pulled before you begin work on a bridge. The waiting time is needed because your gum tissue will shrink at the extraction site. If the bridge is made before the shrinkage is completed, you could have an unsightly space under your bridge. This is more critical for the front teeth than the back teeth.

There are several types of bridges and they each serve a special function. I will stick to the most common type, which 95% of us will use. A bridge is anchored at each end by fitting over teeth which have been filed down, similar to a tooth prepared for a crown. These are called your anchor or abutment teeth. There is a difference in the preparation of a bridge and a crown in that the anchor teeth must be prepared parallel. That is so the bridge can be slipped on several teeth and cemented. If they are not parallel, the bridge will not slip on and the dentist must do a lot of grinding and adjusting to get it to fit.

If you had a bridge put on and it needed a lot of grinding, there is a possibility that the margins of the bridge that fit over the anchor teeth were altered. Have it checked. If you cannot bring your floss down and back up without it catching, then the margins may have been compromised. The problem with this is that you may now have an opening in the margin. This allows bacteria and acid to enter into a less protected part of your tooth and decay will progress faster. This condition can be reduced by having the bridge bonded instead of using regular cement.[13]

You may not notice this condition for years after having your bridge cemented, because the cement itself may fill the space. However, it may wash out over time and then you have the problem to deal with. If you notice this, see your dentist and have it corrected. There are several ways they can treat it. If you catch it quick enough, or have a reasonable dentist, they may not charge you for it if they made the bridge for you. If they do charge you, pay the bill, but consider looking elsewhere for further treatment.

If you are replacing four or more teeth, you may want your bridge anchored on two teeth at each end. Realize it will be more expensive, but it will also be more stable. This can make a big difference depending on your anchor teeth and how long and how healthy the roots are. If they are your eye teeth (also called canine or cuspid teeth) you may get by with only one anchor tooth at each end. I say this because you will put a lot of force on your bridge when you bite, and over a period of time you can cause your anchor teeth to become loose. This will possibly result in more teeth being pulled and a new bridge. If you have four anchor teeth, it will be less of a problem.

When your dentist is grinding down your teeth, if they are alive (vital), ask them to use the water spray. This will keep the tooth cooled down and reduce the possibility of killing the nerve.

An important thing to have included in your bridge is an opening at either end or in-between adjacent teeth that is big enough to insert

---

[13]   Example: All-Bond 2, BISCO Dental Products, www.bisco.com

dental floss through. This opening is called a sluice way and should be on every bridge so you can keep them properly cleaned. Although you now have gold or ceramic over your teeth, they still need to be brushed and flossed. I have seen countless X-rays of patients who have never flossed under their bridges. They have significant bone loss in that area. Some have lost their anchor teeth to periodontal disease. This has meant they now need a larger bridge. When your dentist inserts your bridge, be sure they show you how to use a floss threader and floss under your bridge correctly. It is vital to keep your anchor teeth in good health.

If you lose a porcelain or ceramic facing off of your bridge, it does not mean you need a new bridge. There are new materials that can be bonded to your bridge and still look great. Your dentist should be able to provide it for you with results you like. If they tell you they can't then check around because someone else will.

When you have a porcelain bridge made, get the name of the porcelain used and the color shade or number for your records. If you ever have another bridge made, you may or may not want the same shade. If you know what it was, you'll have a better chance of getting what you want.

If your porcelain bridge comes back from the lab and doesn't match your other teeth or is not the shade you want, talk with your dentist. There is a possibility that some things can be done. They can be tinted right in the office sometimes. They can be sent back to the lab and have the shade changed, but this really depends on how close you are located to the lab and how good the lab is. The important thing is that you should like the results, you're paying for it.

FALSE TEETH

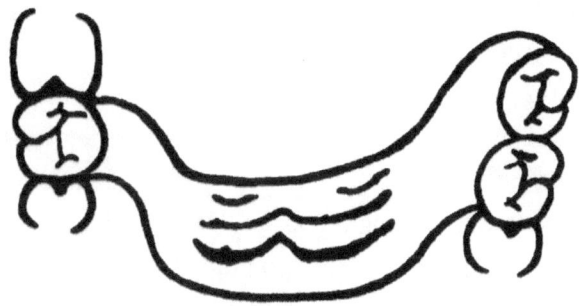

Removable partial dentures serve several functions; they improve appearance, help you chew your food, maintain the space and allow you to keep your remaining teeth. They can last a lifetime if taken care of. You must clean them and your teeth to prevent serious problems.

It is felt by many people that if their parents had dentures, they would also, and they passed that idea on to their children. It has been proven that because your parents or grandparents had dentures, does not mean that you will end up with dentures. If you take care of your teeth, you should be able to break the cycle if you start early enough.

Let's first discuss removable partial dentures or RPD's. These are used when part of your teeth in an arch are missing. There are mostly two types of RPD's used today: those made of metal, and those made of acrylic or plastic.[14] The acrylic RPD's are often called flippers and

---

14 Example: Duraflex Partial Denture, Assured Dental Lab. http://www. assureddentallab.com/

although they can last for years, they are often used as a temporary denture while a metal one is being made or other treatment is being completed. The acrylic RPD's will break easily, so you have to be careful with them. They are not as expensive and can be made in a short time.

The metal RPD's are a more precise partial and more difficult to make. You can expect to see your dentist several times for fittings before they are completed. The advantage with this type of RPD is it will fit better and is much stronger. You also have a wider variety of replacement teeth that can be used.

With either type of RPD you must know one thing. You will most likely experience some rocking motion of your dentures if you have teeth missing only on one side of your mouth. It will be more stable when there are teeth missing on both sides. Your dentist can have clasps put on your denture that will help to hold it in place, however you may have clasps that show when you smile or open your mouth.

With either type of RPD you must wear it and not leave it out of your mouth for long periods of time. If you leave it out for a long period of time you may have your teeth shift. Then your denture will not fit until you have either your teeth or the denture adjusted. Having said that, keep in mind that I'm talking about very long periods of time and not the every night when you need to remove your RPD and put it in a container of water. Your tissue in your mouth needs those nights to be exposed to the air.

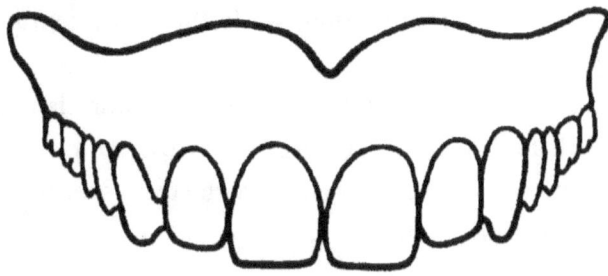

Full dentures can look great and be an improvement to your overall health and self-esteem. Keep them clean and check your gum tissue often for any sores or unusual changes in your gum tissue.

Full dentures, or FD's, will cover your entire arch and replace all your teeth. There is an exception to this rule: when your eye teeth (also called canine or cuspid) are left in place and your FD has two holes in it for those teeth. They will give your denture more stability. These same teeth may also be cut off at the gum line, have root canals done and then fillings placed. They will then support the FD and give them more stability.

Expect to visit your dentist several times in order to have a FD made correctly. There is much more to it than just taking an impression on one visit and inserting a FD on the next visit. You will have impressions, wax try-in's (perhaps several), occlusal registrations and finely your denture, which may also need to be adjusted before you can wear it comfortably. Your dentist may also make an immediate denture for you. The impressions are taken before all your teeth are pulled, wax bite blocks are made and adjusted and then the denture is made and will be inserted during the same appointment that you have your teeth pulled. You will need to visit your dentist again within a few months for checkups and a reline because your gum tissue and supporting bone will shrink after your teeth are removed.

You will find that after wearing your dentures, the upper denture stays in better than the lower. This is not uncommon. The upper denture is often held in by suction, while the lower denture is often held in only by gravity.

FD's are made of acrylic with either plastic or porcelain teeth. The porcelain teeth look better, last longer and cost more. You can also have fillings done on your denture or have the teeth slightly crooked to present a more realistic appearance.

Caring for dentures

In discussing RPD's and FD's what I really want to tell you is how to care for them and yourself. Keep them clean and brush and floss all your remaining teeth daily. When you wear a RPD it creates a food trap and a place for bacteria and plaque to gather between the RPD and your teeth. If you wear a RPD that fits too tightly, have your dentist adjust it because it can cause problems with your remaining teeth. If you develop a sore under your denture, take it out when you notice it and have your dentist adjust your denture if needed. Don't try to adjust it yourself. You can easily make the problem worse or damage your denture. Also, the sore in your mouth needs to be checked to insure you haven't developed a problem. Although you may have full dentures now, you should still have your dentist check your mouth at least once a year just to ensure you are not developing problems you cannot see or feel.

I have a good friend who did not have his denture adjusted or relined when it did not fit well; instead he just kept adding more denture adhesive and wore his denture. This went on for many years until it became painful and the doctors told him he had developed cancer on his pallet under his denture. He had to have most of his pallet and nose removed and plastic surgery to rebuild his face. It is still an on-going problem for him. This illustrates why it is so important for you to see your dentist when you first notice any type of problem. Most dentists will adjust your denture at no cost or little cost if they are the dentist that made the denture for you.

When you go to sleep make sure to take your denture out, clean it and put it in some water. You should do this every day because the tissue in your mouth needs to breathe in order to stay healthy. It cannot do this if your denture is in all the time. When you clean your denture you can use what ever does the job for you, but be careful using abrasives and bleach. They can damage and change the color of your dentures.

Loose dentures

Do not be surprised if you find your denture becoming loose the longer you have it. Often the bone under your gum tissue will absorb or shrink, especially if it is a poor fitting denture. It is important that you are aware of your bone support under your denture. If you lose to much bone, you run the risk of needing extensive surgery to rebuild that bone if, in fact, it can be rebuilt.

If you find that your dentures are loose and need a lot of adhesive to hold them in, your dentist may be able to help you by doing a denture reline. When your dentures will stay in without any adhesive and are comfortable to wear, then you have a denture that is fitted properly. Anything short of that may need further help from your dentist.

One last thing about dentures. For some of you, who wear a metal denture, be aware that your breath may now be more offensive to those around you. People who wear anything like metal dentures and metal orthodontic appliances may have a breath problem that the rest of the population does not have. Keeping your teeth and mouth clean will lessen your chances of offending anyone. Just be aware.

TOOTH SENSITIVITY

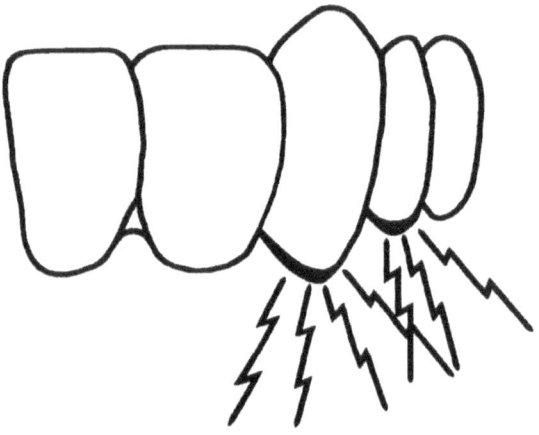

Many who are dedicated to taking care of their teeth develop areas that are very sensitive. Often these areas are near the gum line and if caught quickly, the sensitivity can be eliminated. It does not mean you have decay because your teeth are sensitive.

Many people have tooth sensitivity and the numbers are growing. It may surprise you to learn it is often found in people who are trying to take good care of their teeth and are concerned about them. The cause for a lot of sensitivity might not be what you would think. Would you believe that often you are unknowingly causing it yourself? Some common causes are brushing your teeth incorrectly, using the wrong type of toothbrush, using too much of the wrong type of toothpaste and the misuse of teeth whitening products.

If you are brushing incorrectly, doing it very hard with the wrong type of toothbrush and motion, you may have damaged the gum tissue around the teeth. This tissue will then tend to shrink and after a while, it will shrink enough to expose the root of the tooth. If this happens quickly, your teeth may not have a chance to adapt to the loss of the tissue and they will become sensitive to hot, cold, sweets, and even cold air. If you touch this area with anything, it hurts! Another possible cause for sensitivity is that by brushing too hard and incorrectly, you have removed the outer protective layer on the enamel of your teeth. This is a very thin layer that protects your teeth and keeps them from being so sensitive. Some people who have brushed to hard and removed this layer have teeth that are so sensitive they cannot even breath in cool air through their mouth.

There are treatments that your dentist can do to help. If no decay is involved, they can give you a fluoride treatment on the sensitive teeth. This is a higher concentration of fluoride and not what is used on children's teeth or when you have your teeth cleaned. Another option is to put on a bonding liquid only which seals the tooth and stops the pain. You'll only be able to get these treatments from your dentist. Additionally, you will need to change your brushing technique.

If you are brushing incorrectly with the wrong type of toothbrush you can end up with erosion of your teeth. The more erosion you have the more you have the possibility of sensitivity. Your dentist may treat erosion by the treatments mentioned above or by putting in a bonded filling. If you have lost any gum tissue, there is a composite filling which is pink to help match your gum tissue and it can be used in some but not all cases. If you are brushing your teeth with a hard or medium type of toothbrush, this may be the cause of your sensitivity. I strongly encourage you to try using a soft or extra soft toothbrush and see if there is a difference. You may need to change your brushing habits so you can avoid getting the sensitivity back again.

A leading cause of tooth sensitivity

Surprisingly enough, toothpaste is one of the leading causes of tooth sensitivity. Some contain abrasive ingredients and when used too often and in large quantities they can cause sensitivity to your teeth. We tend to use large amounts of the types that advertise stain removal or whitening of teeth because we are in a hurry to have our teeth white again. If you use these types of toothpaste, use small amounts (about the size of a pea) and don't overdo the brushing. If your teeth start to get sensitive, stop using any toothpaste when you brush and use just a soft or extra soft brush when you brush and let your teeth recover. Teeth that become very sensitive are a bigger problem than when they were not as white as you wanted them to be.

Another possible cause of sensitivity is the self applied teeth whitening (bleaching) treatments. Each time the acid is applied to your teeth, you break down a very small portion of the enamel of your teeth. If this is done too rapidly, you can cause your teeth to become sensitive. If this happens, stop for awhile until the sensitivity is gone, then proceed with caution and be aware of what your teeth are telling you.

Surprising proposed treatment

If you want to stop the sensitivity yourself, try not using any toothpaste at all for a couple of weeks. Brush with only your soft or extra soft toothbrush and use a warm mouthwash with fluoride to freshen your breath. It will take some time, but it may work and save you a trip to the dentist. If it doesn't work, try toothpaste that is made for sensitive teeth. It takes using it for awhile to get the results you want and they may not taste as good, but they will ease your sensitivity. The important thing is to not stop brushing your teeth because they are sensitive; just brush them correctly.

There are other things that cause sensitivity. Chewing hard things like ice and hard candy can do this. Eating too many foods and drinks with high acid content such as citrus fruits and sodas can also contribute. With each of these things, it is simply a matter of changing your habits and giving your teeth time to adjust. If the sensitivity does not go away, have your dentist check for a defective filling or a hairline fracture. They are sometimes hard to detect and can be very painful. If you have one, it means having more work done on your teeth.

CLEANING YOUR OWN TEETH

It use to be that cleaning your own teeth was not a problem, but with a few dental instruments now available to the public, more injuries are occurring. It is not impossible to clean your own teeth with a cleaning (scaling) instrument. I do my own sometimes, but I'm also a trained hygienist. I'm sure there are many dentists and hygienists that clean their own teeth. However if you are not trained, you can hurt yourself or someone else if you try to clean their teeth. You can very easily get an instrument wedged between your teeth and damage them trying to get it out. You can also gouge or scratch the surface of your teeth and cause permanent damage. Perhaps the easiest thing to damage is your gum tissue or the membrane tissue around each tooth. While it will heal in time, you can go through a lot of pain and it could lead to more severe and permanent problems.

I strongly discourage you from trying but if you think you have to clean your teeth, don't try to clean anything below the gum line and be very careful between your teeth. Some of the damage could cost you more to repair than you will ever save by doing it yourself.

Another thing you will miss out on in trying to clean your own teeth is you will miss out on having the dentist or hygienist check all your mouth and letting you know if there is decay or other problems starting.

I had a patient who cleaned his teeth with a paper clip. He had very little tartar (calculus) but he did have some bad scratches and grooves on his teeth. He would have been better off seeing a hygienist and then taking good care of his teeth so he would not develop the tartar and stain. You can aid the prevention of tartar and stain by properly brushing and flossing.

TONGUE BRUSHING

Brushing the tongue is a practice that has existed for centuries. It was not always done with a toothbrush, however. People used a device called a tongue scraper and they would scrape their tongues with it. You can still purchase tongue scrapers and they still work very well. However, we are fortunate that we can also do it effectively with a toothbrush.

Do you need to brush your tongue? Yes! Your tongue is an area on which bacteria and other materials build up. If you look in a mirror and see a coating on your tongue (usually white) then you'll see what I mean. If this is left on your tongue it can cut down on your sense of touch and taste. It is also one of the leading contributors to bad breath.

To get rid of this coating, brush your tongue when you brush your teeth. Brush as far back as the coating goes or as far back as you can without gagging yourself. With continued effort, you'll be able to brush farther back and it will not bother you as much. Once this coating is removed, you can cut down on the amount of time or the frequency of your brushing but don't stop completely.

One advantage of brushing your tongue is that it will help decrease bad breath. It may not eliminate it completely though because there are other contributors to bad breath. Another advantage is that you will be able to taste your food better.

If you have brushed your tongue for a long time (a month or longer) and still have a coating that doesn't change or gets worse, you need to see your dentist and have it evaluated. You may have some problems that only they can help you with. Don't put it off!

MAINTAINING THE SPACE

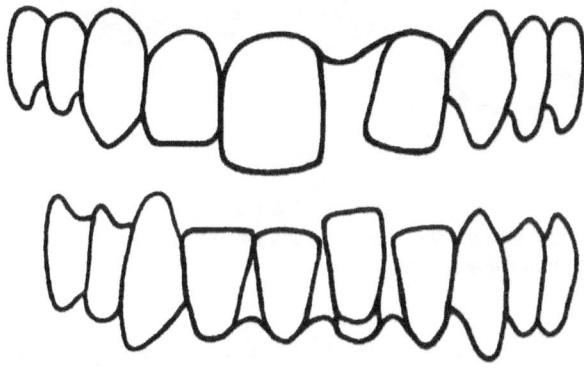

When you loose a front tooth and do not replace it, the other teeth drift forward and fill the space. The opposing tooth may grow into the empty space left when a tooth is pulled and nothing is put there to fill the space.

When a tooth is pulled or knocked out, two things happen: the teeth adjacent to the one pulled will tend to drift into the open space, and if enough space is available, the teeth above/below the one pulled will tend to grow into that vacant space.

If your teeth drift into the vacant space and the missing tooth was a front tooth, you will alter your normal appearance. This can also throw off your bite. Your front teeth will drift forward easier than your back teeth because they do not lock themselves in naturally. Your back teeth can sometimes lock themselves in and may drift very little, if your teeth are not worn flat. When your teeth drift forward, you will need orthodontics to open the space so a false tooth can be placed.

If you are missing several teeth and do not replace them for quite some time with false teeth, you run the risk of having the opposing teeth grow into the vacant space. This can cause you to lose those teeth if you decide later to get false teeth because there will be no room left for the false teeth.

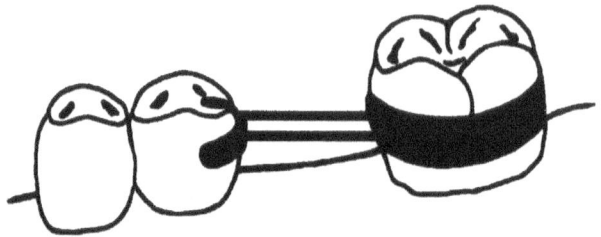

For children, after loosing a tooth if there is some time left before another tooth will grow in, have your dentist place a space maintainer of some type to maintain the vacant space.

If you are young enough to still have teeth that will grow in, have your dentist make a space maintainer of some type for you. This will keep your teeth from drifting and give the tooth space enough to grow. If you have all your teeth and loose one of them, have your dentist make you a partial or a bridge. Get something to maintain the space. Don't wait for your teeth to drift because then you will need orthodontics to move them back or risk loosing more of them in order to have your teeth fixed. If you do nothing, you may pay a heavy price for it later. The odds are really against you.

SEALANTS

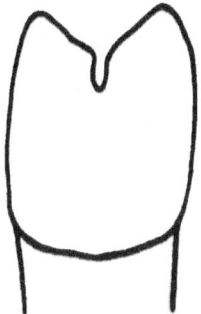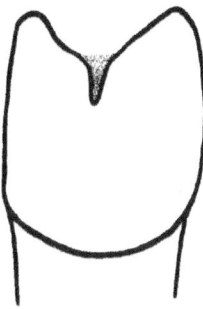

Many of our back teeth have pits or fissures where decay can easily start. Having a pit and fissure sealant used on your children can help prevent decay in their back teeth. It is applied quickly and painlessly.

Parents may want to look at this closely and consider it for their children. The reason for using a sealant is because the anatomy of the back teeth (molars and bicuspids) is made of high and low places formed by different angles coming together. Where these angles come together in the low places, they create what is called a pit or a fissure. These pits and fissures are often too small to get your toothbrush into. Consequently, you have an area for food and bacteria to form and begin their destruction on the enamel of your teeth. This is usually one of the first areas to get decay.

When you notice new teeth coming into the back of your child's mouth (usually 2 to 4 teeth) go to your dentist and have those teeth evaluated for having sealants done. If sealants are done, they will use a technique that will put a composite or resin into those pits and fissures that will adhere to the tooth. This prevents bacteria from occupying that space and causing decay. The procedure does not take long and is painless. Have it checked each time they are in for a checkup, or at least annually, because sealants can be worn off or in rare cases dislodged which would then need to be replaced.

In the past this procedure could only be done on a tooth that never had decay in it. If you had a filling in the tooth, it didn't work. However, because of the advanced technology we now have, materials can be bonded to both the enamel and the filling material. So it would still be an advantage for your child to have each of their back teeth sealed. This procedure should be done on your child until they are old enough to develop good, sound hygiene habits that will keep their teeth clean enough to avoid decay.

IMPLANTS

Dental implantation is one of the more exciting areas of dentistry and many dentists are eagerly taking training so they can participate in it.[15] It is not however, a new area of dentistry. It has been around for years but it has had mixed results and until recently, many were unsatisfactory. Often the body would reject the devices that were implanted.

The good news is that there have been many new materials and techniques devised which greatly improve the chances for success with implants. One of the biggest is help from digital imaging which will give your dentist more of a multidimensional view of your mouths bone structure.[16] This helps them prepare the site for the implant with much more accuracy. This helps to reduce complications and also improves your chances for a successful implant.

Another advantage is that there are new materials that can be used to build up areas where the jaw bone is not thick enough to support an implant. This gives those with advanced periodontal disease the possibility of replacing the bone that was destroyed. Also, for those who have worn dentures for many years and now have very small or narrow jaw bones, it can be built up and with implants they can have a denture or bridge that will be much more stable.

---

[15] Example: Titanium posts (implants) with integrated ball-tops, BioHorizons, (www.biohorizons.com)

[16] Example: PaX Trio, Vatech, www.vatechamerica.com

A personal experience

May I take the liberty of relating the dental history of a dear friend of mine who is currently undergoing treatment for implants. Her name is Joan and in her youth her parents never took her to a dentist. Both of her parents had dentures in their 30's and she felt she just inherited bad teeth. She remembers walking home from school in the winter time and being afraid to inhale with her mouth open because it hurt so much. When she finally did see a dentist, she had decay in every tooth in her mouth. About 20 years ago she was tired of repeatedly going in and having her teeth worked on and asked her dentist to just pull all of them and give her dentures. The dentist told her it is much better to keep her own teeth, she had good gums and the roots looked pretty good also. So she decided to spend the time and expense of having one root canal after another. This cost her many thousands of dollars and a lot of pain. Then her root canals started decaying and she had to have those teeth pulled. One of the reasons for her teeth going bad is that she had dry mouth caused by having chemo therapy and radiation when she had breast cancer. Her dentist suggested that she now have a denture. Her top teeth were pulled and a denture was made. However she could not keep it in because of her dry mouth. Another dentist put 6 posts in her upper gums and 6 holes in her denture. This did help her but it became such a mess to deal with. Her denture would stay in but it never felt comfortable to her. She had to take it out whenever she ate because food would always get under her denture.

Joan and her family moved to a new town and she found a new dentist. She wanted to get her lower 10 teeth removed and a denture made. She also had to have her upper denture repaired often at a cost of $1,000. each time. She asked her new dentist what she should do now. He suggested that she come to a clinic in a distant town where there were many mentors and students like him and have implants done.[17] Because this would be a teaching situation and he would be doing the work himself with the assistance of a full team, he could save her a great deal of money. On her first visit the 6 posts were removed and her upper jaw was rebuilt and a sinus lift done as well as having 9 implants placed up inside her gums. She then had to wait for 9 months to make sure her body would not reject the new bone material and the implants. Her denture was adjusted to fit over the implants for the 9 months she had to wait. She also had to return to the clinic and have 4 implants done on her lower jaw. Joan is currently in that 9 month waiting period, but is healing very well so far. If all goes well after 9 months, they will insert new teeth that never have to be taken out. The good dentist that did this for her saved her over $20,000. by doing this in a teaching setting.

Joan was eager to share her experience and said she would be delighted if it could help anyone avoid the pain and expense she has had over her lifetime.

I am not experienced with implants to any great extent, so I will not give you any comments on which type to go with. I will suggest that if you are thinking about implants, you should talk with others who have them and see what their results have been. Implants will be a big investment so find a dentist that has been doing them for a while or at least one you trust, and have all your questions answered. If the dentist cannot answer all of your questions satisfactorily, go to someone else until you feel comfortable that you've received all the information you are looking for.

Another important thing is that even though you may go for this type of treatment, you must still keep it clean with proper brushing and flossing or you will lose it, just like you can your natural teeth. This type of treatment is not a quick fix to having your teeth replaced. It takes a long time to have it completed, just like in Joan's case. Find out how long it will take up front and consider everything before you go with it.

---

[17] Example: The White Cap Institute, www.whitecapinstitute.com

MOUTH GUARDS

Many of you will have need of a device called a mouth guard. It is always advised for those who participate in sports; especially contact sports such as boxing, hockey, basketball and football. Your dentist can make one for you or if you want a less expensive one you can pick one up at sporting goods stores and fit it at home by following the instructions. If you are careful when you fit it, it can work very well but you must follow directions. Weekend athletes should consider using one.

There is another type of mouth guard that is used most often for teeth grinding and TMJ (Temporomandibular Joint) problems. These problems may be related because those who grind their teeth often have TMJ problems.

A mouth guard provides something for teeth grinders to grind on without wearing down their teeth. This can help reduce the sensitivity caused by grinding your teeth. A mouth guard will open your mouth slightly; which can relax the TMJ and thus reduce some of the discomfort in the TMJ. Mouth guards must be kept clean and you should brush and floss your teeth before wearing one. Mouth guards will need to be replaced occasionally because they are made of resin (plastic) material and can be worn out with the constant grinding.

For a mouth guard used by a tooth grinder or someone with a TMJ problem, you need to see a dentist. They will take an impression of your teeth and have the mouth guard made in a lab. You will usually receive it and have it adjusted at another appointment. It is an excellent way to treat the above problems and may be tried before more extensive and expensive types of treatment are tried.

INFECTION CONTROL

Infection control is something to be aware of before you choose your dentist. It is important because you are the one in the chair.

This subject is receiving a lot of interest and is in the forefront of dentistry. Many dental publications will have an update on infection control. A good dentist should be aware of what is current.

With the concern about contagious diseases like AIDS and hepatitis, cleanliness is a necessity. Besides cleanliness, there are barrier techniques and infection control procedures. For those who have no idea what that is, it is doing everything necessary to prevent the spread of infectious disease and the bacteria or viruses that cause them. This has been helped by OSHA (Occupational Safety and Health Administration). As of March 6, 1992, OSHA has put requirements on the dental profession for infection control. Many of the requirements will affect only the dentists and their staff, but some will also affect you as a patient. As a minimum, dentists and their treatment staff must wear examination gloves, face masks, protective eye wear, and fluid resistant clothing. Some dentists will go farther by wearing a second pair of gloves, and a face shield. So don't be alarmed if they do, it is to protect you both.

There are many styles of clothing worn and no particular style is dictated by the OSHA regulations, although some are suggested. Another reason for dentists and their assistants to wear protective gear is to protect you in case they have anything, even a cold or sore throat. This protects you.

If your dentist is not doing the minimum requirements and it makes you feel uncomfortable, you may want to reconsider letting them work on you. If they are not following this portion of the requirements, what are they doing about the rest? Additional requirements include instruments used in your mouth must be sterilized in a heat or heat-pressure sterilizer, not a liquid. My preference is to have instruments bagged as well, unless they are kept in a separate room until needed.[18] I also prefer the instruments to not be taken out of their bags until I am seated in the room, so that I can see what type of sterilization is being used. There are many variations of sterilization and what your dentist prefers, so if you are concerned be sure to ask.

Times are changing

Many years ago it was common practice to wipe the handpiece and instruments off with alcohol and use them again. We cannot do that now, not with the possibility of AIDS and hepatitis as great as it is. Handpieces are made to be and must be sterilized. If the handpieces are cleaned according to the manufacturers' instructions, they should be ok. If you are worried about whether the handpiece has been cleaned well enough because of suck-back, ask your dentist. Dental units made since 1985 have a one way valve that prevents suck-back. Those made prior to that time can have a one way valve installed. Most dentists should have this problem taken care of, but ask anyway. Again, it's you in the chair.

Additional things to be aware of include cross contamination and barrier techniques. Make sure that if the dentist is working on you and they have to touch something else, (like supplies, equipment, telephone, pencils, etc.) they take their gloves off. They should throw them away and put on a clean pair when they start working on you again. They may also wear over gloves which they put on over their gloves, do what they were going to do and then take them off before they return to work on you. The bottom line is that the dentist does

---

[18]   Example: Defend   Plus   Sterilization   Pouch,   MYDENT INTERNATIONAL, www.mydent.com

not put gloves into your mouth that have touched anything that may be contaminated by someone or something else.

The equipment must also be cleaned between each patient. If you are lucky you will have a dentist that has their equipment covered with plastic which is changed between each patient. The plastic can reduce the cleaning time because it is discarded. If not, the equipment needs to be cleaned and sprayed with a disinfectant. These disinfectants require a 1 to 10 minute wait to disinfect, then they need to dry or be wiped dry. If you are concerned then ask your dentist if they are disinfecting the treatment rooms between patients.

Why is infection control so important? Each time a dentist uses their high speed handpiece, they are shooting an aerosol that contains bacteria and viruses from 5 to 7 feet into the air. This does not stay in the air forever; it lands everywhere. Each time they touch something new they spread germs. You have no idea what the patients before you may have had and you should expect the dentist to protect you the best that they can.

HOW TO PICK A DENTIST?

The question is often asked about how to pick a dentist. Here are several suggestions you may want to consider. Get your telephone book or go on line to see what dentists are available and what their specialties are in your area. Get a recommendation from your previous dentist if they know any one in that area. The most widely used method is to ask around. Talk with neighbors, friends, relatives, and associates. If you know any hygienists or dental assistants, ask them. They usually know several dentists in the area and something about the quality of their work.

It is suggested that you pick someone who belongs to the American Dental Association or the State Dental Association. These are good guides but don't exclude someone because they don't belong. Membership in these associations is expensive and some choose not to pay the added cost. That certainly does not mean they are less qualified or that their work does not meet standards. Many very good dentists do not belong and to the best of my knowledge it is not required.

Should you call 1-800 DENTIST and have them tell you which dentist to go to? If you want to, go ahead. I've heard of emergency situations where they were called and their service was outstanding. It is especially useful after normal hours and on weekends.

There was a dentist who had the reputation of being the best in town because he had a closed practice and took very few new patients. He was also the most expensive dentist in town. Did this make him the best? That is strictly up to you as a patient. This dentist was good, but so were many others and they were more affordable and accepted new patients. They were also more available to help in an emergency situation. It is very hard to label one dentist as the best unless of course they are the only one.

Another dentist I worked with said a dentist needed to have at least 7 to 10 years of experience to know what they were doing. There is no disputing that experience is valuable. However, every dentist will not start their first practice with that type of experience unless they were in the military, worked for a government agency, HMO or something similar. There are some very good new dentists and many of them are more acquainted with the newer methods and materials being used. So if you find a new dentist and feel good about them, give them a chance.

If you are told something by the dentist you picked and it doesn't seem right to you, question it. Then do what you would do if a physician told you something and you didn't feel right about it. Get a second opinion.

One thing to look for in picking a dentist is how clean their office and treatment rooms are. If they are not cleaned up to your standards, leave. Consider the level of infection control. Also don't be mislead into thinking that because a dentist has a new office or equipment that it makes them a good dentist. Every dentist can have the same equipment. It depends on how much they want to spend. What counts is what they do to you, how you are treated and what you walk out with. I've had great work done by dentists with older equipment and I'd go back to them again if I needed to.

Again, remember what I said earlier. You are not locked into one dentist. If there is anything about them or their staff you don't like, then talk with them about it or change dentists. If they want you as a patient, they will do their best to keep you happy and satisfied.

DENTAL SPECIALISTS

Let me give you a very brief description of the specialists in dentistry. This may help you decide which type you will need if the occasion arises.

Orthodontist: This dentist treats the many types of malocclusions in the mouth. Mostly they will straighten teeth and correct your bite. Many in this specialty will also work with the TMJ (Temporomandibular Joint). For those who have never thought about it, this specialist also helps restore self-esteem in people who are ashamed of the way their teeth look. I've seen fantastic work done in this area. My wife and all of our children have had orthodontic work done, with great results.

Endodontist: This dentist will primarily perform root canals and related treatments. They specialize in the very difficult root canals that other dentist don't want to attempt. I've just finished seeing one and his treatment was great.

Periodontist: This dentist will primarily perform periodontal treatments. This will include root planning, gingivectomy, laser surgeries and full flap procedures with bone reduction, contouring and transplants. They can sometimes help you regenerate some of the bone and soft tissue you have lost. Many in this specialty are also doing implants.

Prosthodontist: This dentist will primarily be involved with the making of prosthetics (false teeth). This will include the making of crowns, bridges, onlays, inlays, removable partials and full dentures. Many in this specialty are also doing implants.

Pedodontist: This is a very courageous dentist. I can't say enough about them and the very important role they play because this is the one that specializes in treating children. They are especially good for children with disabilities. If your child has any type of a disability I highly recommend you see this type of dentist. This dentist could set your child's dental attitude for the rest of their lives.

Oral Surgeon: This dentist is the one who gets the difficult work. They do difficult extractions; the ones that other dentists feel they cannot handle. They repair broken jaws. They also do very sophisticated surgery such as the reduction of the upper and lower jaws and repositioning of the teeth and bone. I've seen beautiful work done by these doctors. One did a lot of work on my son after a bad accident. I'll be forever grateful to him. If you ever read this book Pat, thank you!

General Practitioners: This is also a specialty just like the others and requires additional time and training. These dentists receive more in depth training in many areas of dentistry and can work in the specialties to a much greater extent than regular dentists.

All of these specialists have taken the time, made personal sacrifices, and paid a lot of money for the extended training and education needed for their specialty. In most cases, it is at least two years of training and education beyond dental school. In addition, there are continuing education courses and seminars that they must take to keep their license and be current in their chosen specialty. Believe me, when you need them you are glad they were willing to make the sacrifices necessary to be where they are. Be ready to pay the higher cost associated with using their expertise and skill. They earned it.

You will also find in your search for a specialist that there are many GPs that will specialize in one or two particular areas. That is, they have a particular interest in this area and have chosen to focus on it along with keeping their general practice. Many are very good at their chosen area even though they may not be board certified.

ABOUT THE AUTHOR

The author has over 20 years of dental experience. He received the majority of his training in the United States Air Force. Serving as a dental assistant, expanded functions dental assistant, and a dental hygienist. After retiring from the military he then spent the next 7 years working with civilian dentists and dentists in state institutions. He and his wife of 44 years are currently retired and trying to live the good life with family and friends.

GLOSSARY

Abrasion Wearing away of the hard surface of your teeth by grinding your teeth or by repeatedly using something abrasive on them.

Abscess In dentistry an infection in a localized area of the gum tissue *(gingiva)* or the root tip *(apex)* of a tooth. Usually pus will be present with a light yellow or white color.

Abscess, periapical An infection localized at the tip of a root. Usually very painful and necessary for antibiotics to be used. Most of the time a root canal must be done or pull the tooth.

Abscess, periodontal An infection localized in an area of the gum tissue adjacent to your tooth. Usually painful and necessary for antibiotics to be used. Usually treated with a deep scaling, oral hygiene instruction, nutritional counseling, and rest instructions.

Abutment A tooth, root (after a root canal), or implant used for the support of a bridge or partial denture.

Acrylic The type of resin used for the construction of dental appliances such as partials, full dentures and night guards.

Acute Necrotizing Ulcerative Gingivitis *(ANUG)* A painful, progressive infection of the gum tissue *(gingiva)*.

AIDS Acquired Immunodeficiency Syndrome.

Alloy *(amalgam)* Most dental alloys have silver, tin, copper and zinc in different ratios and are mixed with mercury so they can be molded into the tooth cavity.

Anatomy In dentistry, the art of restoring the appearance and function of a tooth.

Anesthetic A drug that makes your mouth numb so that you loose both feeling and sensation of pain.

Anterior teeth The upper *(maxillary)* and lower *(mandibular)* front teeth (incisors and cuspids).

Antibiotic A medication which is able to stop and destroy bacteria and other microorganisms.

Apex The end of the tooth root.

Appliance A device used to provide function such as a partial or space maintainer.

Base The thin layer of medication or cement that serves as an insulator and protective barrier under a restoration.

Bicuspid The two teeth located forward of the molar teeth. Also called a *Premolar.*

Bleaching The use of chemical agents to lighten discolored teeth.

Bonding The chemical action of securing one substance to another substance. Bonding may be used for composites, alloys, crowns, bridges and orthodontics.

Bridge A prosthetic device consisting of artificial teeth *(pontic)* that are cemented to abutment teeth.

Broach An instrument with barbs sticking out from a metal shaft. Used in root canal *(endodontic)* treatment to remove the nerve from the tooth.

Calculus *(Often called tarter)* A very hard deposit that attaches to the teeth.

Canal The pulp chamber of a tooth located in the root.

Cavity A hole in a tooth usually caused by decay.

Cementum The substance covering the root surface of the tooth.

Ceramics Dental restorations made from fused porcelain.

Clasps The attachments of a partial denture or space maintainer that grasp the natural teeth.

Composite A tooth colored material made of resins use primarily for filling front teeth.

Contour To make a filling to have the shape and form of the original tooth.

Crown The portion of your tooth that is covered with enamel. The cast restoration that covers the portion of your tooth that was covered with enamel.

Curettage Scraping or cleaning away of diseased tissue with an instrument called a curette.

Cusp A pointed or rounded surface of a tooth.

Cuspid (*Also called the canine or eye teeth*) The front tooth next to the incisors with the long thick root.

Decay (*Caries*) A disease that destroys your teeth.

Decalcification The early breakdown of a tooth's enamel by acids found in plaque and other sources, not yet full blown decay. Its appearance is dull and chalky.

Dental floss A thread like material, often made of nylon, used to remove plaque and debris from between your teeth.

Dental hygienist A licensed preventive oral health professional who primarily cleans teeth and teaches you how to take care of your own teeth.

Dentin The inner portion of the tooth below the enamel and over the pulp. Not as hard as enamel and will decay much faster.

Denture A prosthetic substitute for missing teeth. May be complete (full) or partial.

Disclosing solution A tablet or liquid solution that when put on your teeth will stain plaque and show you where you need to brush.

Disinfectant An agent used to kill germs but not necessarily sterilizing the material.

Enamel The very hard tissue that covers the crown of the tooth.

Erosion The wearing away of your teeth but not usually by bacteria.

Eruption The moving of a tooth into its natural position in the mouth.

Etch Treating enamel with phosphoric acid to provide retention for sealants, composite materials, or orthodontic brackets.

Etchant The acid solution or gel used to etch tooth enamel.

Eugenol A liquid obtained from clove oil and other natural sources, usually used as a sedative.

Exposure Exposing the pulp by going through the dentin and into the pulp chamber.

Extraction To pull a tooth.

File A metal instrument with ridges or teeth on its cutting surfaces. Can be small and used for a root canal or larger and used to remove an overhang.

Fissure A deep groove on the top surface of the back teeth.

Fistula An abnormal canal *(tract)* from an internal cavity, or tooth root, through hard and soft tissue to another area or surface.

Floss threader A device often made of plastic or wire that is used to thread dental floss under a dental bridge.

Flossing aid A plastic device that will hold your dental floss and allows you to floss all the necessary surfaces of all your teeth without putting your fingers in your mouth. Great when flossing someone else's teeth.

Fluorosis Spotted enamel caused by excessive fluoride intake.

Gingivectomy The removal of excess gum tissues (gingiva) that does not extend into the underlying bone.

Gingivitis Inflammation of the gum tissues *(gingiva)* characterized by changes in color, appearance, bleeding, and sometimes pus. Also known as Type I periodontal disease.

Gums (*gingiva*) The tissue which immediately surrounds a tooth and is continuous with its periodontal ligament and with the mucosal tissues of the mouth.

Incipient decay The beginning stages of decay that have not broken through the enamel and into the dentin of a tooth.

Incisor Front *(anterior)* teeth with thin and sharp cutting edge.

Infection control Doing everything necessary to prevent the spread of infectious disease and bacteria or viruses that cause them.

Inlay A cast restoration usually gold or ceramic prepared outside the mouth and cemented in a preparation that is designed to restore one, two, or three surfaces of the tooth.

Leakage When any fluid is capable of getting between a restoration and the surrounding tooth structure.

Malocclusion When the teeth in the upper and lower jaws do not come together correctly.

Margin In cavity preparations, the outside edge of the preparation.

Maxillary arch The teeth in the upper jaw.

Molar A back *(posterior)* tooth with a broad top *(occlusal)* surface for chewing.

Mouth guard An acrylic (hard or soft) appliance made on a mold of a persons teeth and used to protect the teeth or prevent teeth grinding.

Occlusal The chewing surfaces of the back *(posterior)* teeth.

Occlusion The contact between the top *(maxillary)* and lower *(mandibular)* teeth in all movements.

Occlusal registration Movements of the jaw that are marked and recorded by the dentist so that when a denture is made the same movements will be duplicated when wearing the denture.

Onlay A cast restoration usually of gold or ceramic prepared outside the mouth and designed to restore two or more cusps of the occlusal surface of a back *(posterior)* tooth.

Overhang Excess restorative material projecting over the cavity margin. Needs to be removed as soon as possible.

Palatal Area involving the palate, or roof of the mouth.

Partial denture Prosthetic device containing artificial teeth on a framework of resin or metal and attaches to natural teeth by means of metal clasps.

Periapical abscess An abscess at the apex or root end of a tooth.

Periodontal abscess An abscess in bone and/or gum tissue surrounding a tooth.

Periodontal scaling and root planing The procedure designed to remove the tarter *(calculus)* and diseased tissue on the root surface of a tooth in the pockets around your teeth.

Periodontal ligament The tissues that support and anchor the tooth in its socket.

Periodontal pocket The area around the root of a tooth that has lost the bone support due to tarter (calculus) being left over a long period of time and not removed.

Pit and fissure Enamel that during formation resulted in very narrow depressions in the chewing surface. These should be sealed to prevent decay.

Plaque A soft deposit on the teeth consisting of bacteria, sugars, acids and food debris. A primary cause of tooth decay.

Posterior teeth The upper *(maxillary)* and lower *(mandibular)* back teeth, bicuspids and molars.

Premolar A bicuspid tooth with points and cusps for grasping, tearing, and chewing.

Pulp chamber The inside portion of your tooth that contains the nerves and blood vessels.

Pulp capping To place a medication over the pulp when exposed or nearly exposed during a cavity preparation.

Pus A thick fluid often light yellow to white in color that can be found at the site of an infection.

Recession When you loose part of your gum tissue over the root of your tooth.

Retention The act of making something stay in place, this can be done with mechanical locking or bonding.

Root canal The removal of the pulp chamber (nerves and blood vessels) of a tooth and then having the pulp chamber filled with a filling material and then sealed.

Scaling The physical removal of the plaque and tarter *(calculus)* from the surface of the crown and root of a tooth.

Sealant A bonding material that is used to fill up pits and fissures to prevent decay from getting started.

State Dental Practice Act Each state has laws that control what a dentist and their dental staff are allowed to do.

State Board of Dental Examiners They interpret and implement those regulations contained in the State Dental Practice Act. If you have a serious problem with a dentist or their staff and cannot resolve it, this is who you contact.

Sterilization The process of destroying all forms of life on a designated item or in a designated area.

Suck-back The liquid that is sucked back into a dental handpiece from a patient's mouth at the moment a dentist stops using the handpiece.

Sulcus The area around a tooth where the gum tissue is not attached to the surface of the tooth. In a healthy mouth this can be from 1 mm to 3 mm in depth.

Super eruption When a tooth continues to grow into the vacant space on the opposing arch where a tooth has been removed.

Tarter *(calculus)* A very hard deposit that attaches to the teeth. Has its beginning as plaque.

Temporary filling Material (often medicated) placed in a tooth to sedate the tooth and calm it down so that it can be worked on with less chance of killing the nerve. Also to occupy space and protect the tooth until the tooth can be worked on or completed.

Veneer A very thin tooth colored material that is bonded to the front surface of your front teeth. Usually made of porcelain or composite. Often used to hide badly broken down teeth or badly stained teeth.

Water irrigation device A device that allows you to shoot water under adjustable amounts of pressure into the sulcus or pockets around your teeth to aid in keeping them clean.

INDEX

www.ingramcontent.com/pod-product-compliance
Lightning Source LLC
Chambersburg PA
CBHW051442280526
45785CB00003B/1396